BOOM

STRONG BODY · SHARP BRAIN · ENDLESS ENERGY

Told in a way that both delights and inspires, *Boom: 6 Steps to a Longer, Healthier Life* provides a template to get moving. Cathy's strategies are a great fit for busy executives who want to stay healthy and at the same time, help their organization better integrate well-being in the workplace. Well done! **—Laura Putnam, CEO of Motion Infusion and author of** *Workplace Wellness that Works*

Great job, Cathy! You present a very upbeat "you CAN do it" message. It's apparent that you've been in this industry a long time and have really listened to people. As I read along, I found myself saying "but they will ask....", and every time you were right on it. This book also achieves the purpose of inspiring anyone to really try some form of exercise. You are caring and understanding with regard to failed attempts while inspiring to try again. **—Dan Kolar, Manager, Fitness Facility at Marriott International Headquarters**

A refresher course to get you back on track to doing what you should be doing! Let Cathy guide you to a better you; the best you this year! She tells you the facts and keeps it interesting. **—Laura Cotton RD LD CLC, Austin, TX**

Cathy is a great storyteller who uses practical real-life examples of simple things we can do to be healthier. She motivated ME! I'm sold on her "never too early, never too late" philosophy and have already made changes in my day-to-day habits thanks to Cathy! **—Dotty Raleigh, Middletown, MD**

Need motivation to FINALLY make positive changes to your health and well-being? Resolve to live your best life now by reading *Boom: 6 Steps to a Longer, Healthier Life* by Cathy Richards. This book will show you why exercising is hands down the best prescription for a healthy mind, body and spirit. Follow Cathy's guidelines and your quality of life will increase! —**Peter Colwell, author,** *Spell SUCCESS in Your Life and Invest in Your Attitude,* **www.petercolwell.com**

Cathy provides a compelling message that modest lifestyle changes can yield meaningful results at any age. Her tips and philosophy will go a long way helping all of us to age in a healthier way. —**Jill Vitale-Aussem, President and CEO, The Eden Alternative and author of** *Disrupting the Status Quo of Senior Living: A Mindshift*

Cathy's "never too early, never too late" fitness model provides two separate tracks that highlight important exercises for younger and older adults who don't have a lot of time but want to stay healthy and mobile as they age. Thank you, Cathy! —**Priti Prabhu, board-certified Physical Therapist, Mobility & More, Inc.**

Do yourself a favor and heed Cathy's "don't wait" advice to start focusing on your health and wellness today. She makes a great case for making a wise investment now to be as active as possible later. —**Colin Milner, Founder and CEO, International Council on Active Aging**

Leaders in the senior living industry have much to gain from Cathy's insights on supporting the dual wellness efforts of both team members and the elders they serve. Cathy's blueprint lays the groundwork for building relationships, health, and community all at the same time. **—Dennis Hunter, Vice President, Brooke Grove Foundation**

This book is an inspirational guide for anyone who wants to start now to improve the quality of their health. Many books of this type can be intimidating, but Cathy Richards' tone is encouraging and down-to-earth. As Cathy says, "it's never too late" and because of this I highly recommend it, especially to older adults and their caregivers. **—Jennifer L. FitzPatrick, MSW, CSP, Author,** *Cruising Through Caregiving: Reducing the Stress of Caring for Your Loved One*

IT'S NEVER TOO EARLY AND NEVER TOO LATE!

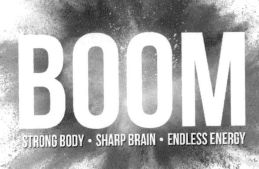

BOOM

STRONG BODY · SHARP BRAIN · ENDLESS ENERGY

6 STEPS to a LONGER, HEALTHIER LIFE

CATHY RICHARDS, M.A.

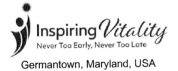

Inspiring *Vitality*
Never Too Early, Never Too Late

Germantown, Maryland, USA

BOOM
6 Steps to a Longer, Healthier Life

ISBN: 978-0-9767800-1-4 (Paperback)
ISBN: 978-0-9767800-2-1 (eBook)

Published by
Fitness InSight/Inspiring Vitality
13402 Queenstown Lane
Germantown, MD 20874
www.CathyRichards.net

The "Never Too Early-Never Too Late Four-Level Exercise Plan" and the corresponding "BOOM Fitness Framework" Exercise Dial are trademarks of Inspiring Vitality/Fitness InSight.

This publication contains the opinions and ideas of its author. Every effort has been made to ensure the accuracy and clarity of the information contained, however, neither the author nor the publisher assume any responsibility for errors, omissions, or changes that occur after publication. This book is sold with the understanding that the author and publisher are not engaged in rendering professional advice or services to the individual reader. The ideas and suggestions in this book are not intended as a substitute for consulting with your physician. The author and publisher specifically disclaim all responsibility for any liability, loss, or risk, personal or otherwise, which is incurred as a consequence, directly or indirectly, of the use and application of any of the contents of this book.

THANK YOU FOR PURCHASING

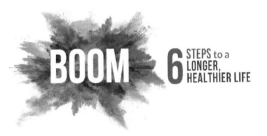

BOOM **6** STEPS to a LONGER, HEALTHIER LIFE

I have two free gifts for you!

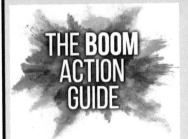

THE **BOOM** ACTION GUIDE

I've created an action guide that you can use to capture your personalized action steps from the book. This tool is the best way to fast-track your progress toward a longer, healthier life with a strong body, sharp brain, and endless energy.

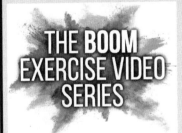

THE **BOOM** EXERCISE VIDEO SERIES

If a picture is worth a thousand words, a video is worth ten thousand words! I can't wait for you to try the exercises outlined in **BOOM**! There are illustrations of each exercise within the book, but to help you even more, I've created video demonstrations showing exactly how to perform each exercise correctly. You'll also find information on how to select and obtain the inexpensive fitness equipment needed for some of the exercise routines.

Access both of your free gifts here:
www.CathyRichards.net/BoomExtras

This book is dedicated to my parents, John and Concetta Schulien. I couldn't ask for more loving or supportive parents or for better examples of active, healthy aging.

This book is also dedicated to my husband Matt, who is always by my side no matter what.

Finally, this book is dedicated to my children Jenna, Jeff, and Matt, and stepchildren Emily, Tyler, and Dylan who keep me guessing and going! Life keeps changing and it's my greatest joy to be part of your lives as you live out your own dreams.

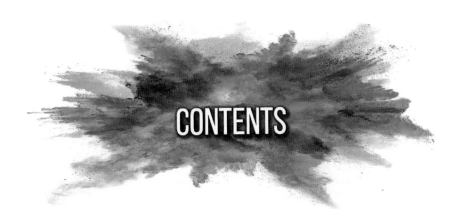

CONTENTS

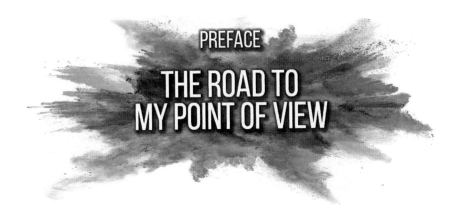

THE ROAD TO MY POINT OF VIEW

I'VE BEEN FASCINATED by the workings of the human body since I was young. As a child, I was also a conscientious rule-follower and a good student. Mix those together and you have the makings of a naturally health-conscious person. I have an early memory of putting grape jelly on my toast instead of cinnamon and sugar, thinking it was healthier; only to find out that jelly is mostly sugar!

As the eldest daughter of five children, I had no problem telling other people what to do. If my parents went out, my mother would tell my older brother to take care of himself and tell me to take care of the rest of the kids. I think I enjoyed being Mom's little helper a little longer than my younger siblings did!

My parents set a great example of making time for fitness, even while raising five children. At the time, I had no idea how difficult it must have been. In addition to driving us to our sports practices, our parents managed to play tennis, racquetball, and volleyball on a regular basis.

My own athletic pursuits were unimpressive. I played softball in elementary school and basketball in middle school and can safely say that I barely touched the ball in either sport. I attended an all girls' high school and was a cheerleader for our neighboring boys' school, with a decidedly nonathletic purpose!

While I was in high school, I had my first exposure to the field that I would ultimately study. My ninth-grade science class was Human Physiology, including the inner workings of the cardiovascular system, the muscular system, and all the other systems of the body. It was co-taught by a science teacher and a P.E. teacher and soon became my favorite class.

I hadn't yet made the connection to daily living but during lunchtime, I would curiously watch that same P.E. teacher running around the campus grounds. I thought it was an odd sight and just shook my head while munching my Doritos. It was my understanding at the time that the only reason to exercise was to participate in sports. To exercise for no reason at all was a new concept to me.

I entered college as a biology major and assumed I'd pursue some type of health or medical career. That's when I experienced pizza delivery for the first time... and proceeded to gain the dreaded "Freshman 15" pounds. As a sophomore, I decided to do something about the weight and signed up for an aerobics class for elective credits. I figured that if I had to go to class, I would lose weight at least.

What I didn't count on was a lecture component to the class in addition to the exercise. The lectures were reminiscent of 9th grade physiology and I was introduced to Kinesiology/Exercise Science as a major. I lost weight, but I gained even more—a new major that I was excited about. Upon graduation, I went on to Graduate School in Exercise Physiology, and brought things full circle by teaching the same undergraduate aerobics class that first excited me as a sophomore. It was a good feeling and gave me the opportunity to teach and mentor hundreds of college students to start early with good health and exercise habits.

While I was still in college, I was fortunate to stumble upon a great job in the corporate fitness center at Marriott International Headquarters. I learned the practical side of the fitness industry— performing fitness tests, teaching people how to use the exercise machines, and teaching group exercise classes.

A corporate fitness center is a different environment than an outside health club in that you spend the full day within the corporate environment. I got to know many busy working professionals and began to understand the difficulty they had fitting exercise into their stressful daily lives. I served on a committee that was planning a comprehensive wellness program and ended up with a new full-time job managing the program. Marriott has always had the philosophy that if you "take care of the associate, they will take care of the customer" and I couldn't think of a better place for me to gain my early wellness career experience. I organized special events such as health fairs, wellness seminars, and team walks, and continued to promote healthy living.

During my fifteen total years at Marriott, I had three children. After my second child was born, I started a part-time personal training business at home and when my third child was born, I left the corporate setting to work exclusively at home with a more flexible schedule. This began my next phase of working with busy moms. Everywhere I went—preschool drop off, the elementary school bus stop, or the grocery store—moms would ask, "How do you fit in exercise?". Practical advice was part of it, but they were also looking for motivation. I wrote *The Busy Mom's Ultimate Fitness Guide: Get Motivated and Find the Solution that Works for You* in order to put all of my suggestions in one place. It was rewarding to help other moms figure out how to fit in fitness and do something for themselves that would also set a good example for their children.

As my children grew, I re-entered the full-time workforce as Director of Fitness and then Director of Lifestyle and Wellness for a large continuing care retirement community, home to over 1,400 older adults with an average age of 85. Although I had extensive experience in wellness, I had very little experience with older adults. It was fantastic and life changing. In my eight years at this community, I met extraordinary, inspiring, active, fun, and funny people. I also met tired, lonely, achy, and unwell people with regrets and lessons to share, and many who fell somewhere in between. The wisdom that comes with age is not a mere cliché and yet the American culture is not one that seems to be noticeably appreciative of it.

The most significant thing I observed in the older adult setting was the huge variation in quality of life, outlook on life, mobility, and both physical and mental health for people who are the same chronological age. I began to wonder what determined the difference. Were the major contributing factors luck, genetics, and/or their *current* lifestyle habits? Or, could it be that their lifestyle habits in *all the decades leading up to* their current age were a major contributor? I noticed patterns and lessons that those of us who are many years younger can benefit from if only we can heed their warning. I felt like Marty McFly in the movie *Back to the Future*, taking lessons learned with the older adults back to my corporate-aged clients to tell them, "I have seen your future! If you aren't living a healthy life yet, start now!"

The second most significant thing I noticed is that the amazing human body can indeed make adaptations at any age. I observed eighty-four and eighty-five-year-olds making noticeable improvements to their health, mobility, and quality of life with just a few small lifestyle changes.

Ever since I wrote and published *The Busy Mom's Ultimate Fitness Guide* in 2006, I've had the idea that I would someday repurpose the material for a broader audience. Many of the concepts I wrote about are applicable to anyone who wants practical advice on fitting in healthy habits. After working with the older adult population and drawing parallels between the varied groups I've worked with, now is the time. I've adapted several sections of this book from my earlier writing and I can't think of a better way to honor the different populations I've worked with than to highlight the benefits and connections of living well at every stage of life.

College students, working adults, busy moms, and older adults have much in common. *It's never too early and it's never too late to make modest lifestyle changes that will yield meaningful improvements to our quality of life.* I have found my professional philosophy and mantra. Let's go!

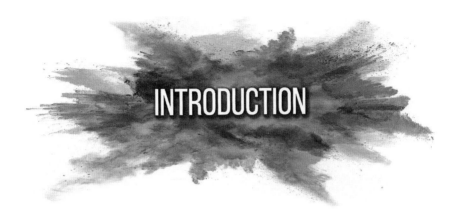

INTRODUCTION

BOOM. Can you think of a time when you felt like life was giving you a wake-up call?

Boom. Are you tired of starting and stopping attempts at healthier habits (or worse—keeping your head in the sand)? Do you want to just DO THIS ALREADY?

Boom. The day you realize you simply can't afford *not* to make some changes.

Boom. Done. Have you ever heard someone use the phrase "Boom. Done." as if an action or success was a foregone conclusion? Are you ready to apply that mindset to your own health and fitness? I hope so because truly, it doesn't have to be hard, complicated, or restrictive. *BOOM* will make you a believer that there really are small habits that deliver big results for your body, brain, and energy level now *and* help you lead a longer, healthier life later.

SIX STEPS TO A LONGER, HEALTHIER LIFE

Are there really only six steps to a longer and healthier life? The skeptic in you should be wary! Of course, there aren't six simple steps to anything far-reaching and worthwhile. In this book, however, I've devised a system to mentally organize important aspects of achieving a longer, healthier life into six steps. Think of each step as a stage or body of knowledge to master. Some steps involve changing how we *think*, while other steps require changing what we *do*. When we successfully alter both our ways of thinking and doing, magic can happen!

STEP ONE:

A STRONG BODY, SHARP BRAIN, AND ENDLESS ENERGY STARTS IN YOUR HEAD

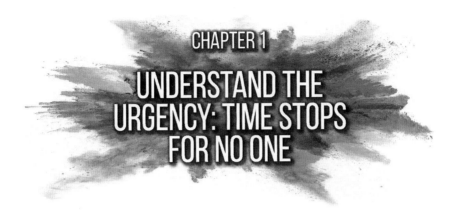

CHAPTER 1

UNDERSTAND THE URGENCY: TIME STOPS FOR NO ONE

" *Isn't it funny how day by day nothing changes, but when you look back, everything is different?*" My son Jeff selected this quote from C.S. Lewis for his senior yearbook to summarize his thoughts on his four years of high school. It was a wise observation that also applies to our health over the years. We might not see the effects of our small, everyday habits now, but after a lifetime of good, bad, or in-between habits, the impact adds up one way or another.

In order to live a longer, healthier life, there are three health goals that will help get you there: a *Strong Body, Sharp Brain, and Endless Energy*. Imagine how it would feel to live that reality every day. Goodbye to aches and pains, a foggy mind, and lethargy. Hello to vitality of mind and body. Combined, these three gems are the key to, quite simply, being able to do what we want to do! Luckily, many of the factors that determine our strength of body and brain, and our energy levels are within our control. In addition, there is tremendous overlap in the strategies that lead to all three, so we don't have to worry about following three different sets of recommendations.

Regardless of your age, the time is now, hence my personal mantra: It's NEVER TOO EARLY and it's NEVER TOO LATE! Once you understand the urgency and then begin to see that it's not as hard or as time-consuming as you thought, you will wonder why you didn't start sooner!

After spending eight years surrounded by over 1,400 people with an average age of 85, I started asking younger populations: What type of 85-year-old do you want to be?

Picture yourself at 85. What do you look like? What pursuits fill your day? How healthy are you? You may not have given this much thought. After all, we live in a society that is focused on youth and the present. We see value placed on immediacy and instant gratification and there is very little attention given to the dutiful and boring applications of advance planning.

> When Jeff was in middle school, he had many neighborhood friends and would run from house to house, seeing which friends were home and when they could play so he could fit them all in. He did great in school, despite having the messiest room and messiest backpack I have ever seen. He had a giant binder exploding with dog-eared papers, all out of order and not even in the prongs. Occasionally, I'd help him clean out his binder, but it was a never-ending cycle. Let's just say that Jeff did not understand the benefit of doing certain things now that would benefit him later.
>
> In high school, Jeff's friendships were still high priority and his jovial aversion to planning was still the same. While doing homework, he would prop up his phone in "Facetime" mode every night and his laughter filled the house into the wee hours. He had a separate binder for each subject, which meant he now had seven binders that were a mess. He still left everything to the last minute. One day when I was nagging him about being more organized, he gave me a huge grin and said, "Mom, that's future Jeff's problem." He was absolutely serious! (I didn't find out until later

that it was a line from a popular sitcom!) It became his standard answer to all questions regarding boring tasks that could be put off until some vague future time. My standard response was "Please think about future Jeff!" Thankfully, although these habits continued through all of high school, Jeff still did well and earned a Naval ROTC scholarship to Purdue. Off he went to college, with my fingers crossed.

Jeff's first year at Purdue didn't exactly go smoothly. The demands of ROTC combined with the rigors of his academics meant that the workload has finally reached a capacity at which Jeff's habits began to fail him. There were a few learning lessons like oversleeping and missing his ROTC early morning workout. Or, waking up in time for the workout, but coming home and sitting down for "a minute" only to fall back asleep with an apple in his hand and missing a major presentation. He had to retake the entire class. The consequences were stacking up, causing him to rethink some of his habits. He called me and said, "Mom, did you know that there's an alarm on my phone? I can set it if I need to be someplace." "Also, I hung a calendar above my desk and I was thinking that I could start writing down due dates for tests and big projects." and finally "Mom, if there's something I need to do in the future, I can just write it down on a list and keep the list with me." It was all I could do to resist telling him that I had already suggested all of these things in the past! Present Jeff began to care deeply about future Jeff's problems and things began to improve from that point on.

Let's return to the question, "What type of 85-year-old do you want to be?"

Younger people don't usually contemplate what life will be like when they are 85, much less that what they are doing today will have any bearing on it. When you are 25, you think you are going to live forever; 35, raising a young family; 45, gunning your career to the top; 55, starting to joke about aging aches and pains; and 65, perhaps starting to think about life at 85 because you might be caring for your own aging parent.

The reason I continue to pose this question to younger adults is that regardless of your current age, you are working toward your 85-year-old self *right now*, for better or for worse. Is your quality of life at the age of 85 your *future self's* problem or are you willing to take ownership of it now? Are you like the old Jeff or the new Jeff? Are you keeping your binders neat all along, or are you banking on periodic clean-up sessions that may or may not be successful because some of the papers are lost or damaged beyond repair? Many of us "get by" in our younger years without great habits, just like Jeff did in middle school and high school, but by our older years, the consequences start adding up, as they did for Jeff in college.

The years are flying by. In fact, at almost every age, people wonder and joke out loud, "How did I get this old?" We think we are "old" at 30, then 40, then 50, and then in future years, we WISH we could be "that young" again. Can you remember how you felt 20 years ago? Did that time go by quickly? What age will you be 20 years from now? Won't those 20 years go by just as quickly—if not more so? Don't wait! Think about *thriving* through the years!

While I worked in senior living communities, I met thousands of 85-year-olds, some with significant physical and cognitive ailments and serious challenges in daily living that made it difficult to enjoy their lives. I met other 85-year-olds who were finding much more satisfaction in life in whatever way they defined it—finding new loves, participating in competitive sports, or traveling the world! What is the biggest determinant of the difference? It's not luck, genetics, or your habits at the age of 84.

The largest determinants of your health at the age of 85 are your lifestyle habits in the decades leading up to that age—your twenties, thirties, forties, fifties, sixties, and seventies.

John Rowe and Robert Kahn's *MacArthur Foundation Study of Successful Aging in America* gave us the gifts of optimism and control over how we age. We know that life expectancy is increasing but living longer doesn't mean those additional years are necessarily quality years. While certainly not everything that can befall us as we age is within our control, their research tells us that we don't need to anticipate aging as an inevitable period of total decline. Rowe and Kahn went even further to show us that in fact, **up to 70% of how we age is determined by lifestyle!** There is much we can do through our lifestyle to *preserve* our health, mobility, and quality of life, and even *improve* it as we age.

Look at the graph below from Rowe and Kahn's book *Successful Aging.* The solid line shows a gradual decline in physical and cognitive functioning starting at middle age. Not a pleasant thought about aging, is it? Look at the dotted line as an alternative model for aging. Notice how this style of aging includes maintaining close to 100% of our functioning capacity much farther into older age, before experiencing some type of health setback (the "blip" on the dotted line) that leads to a much later but quicker descent. My mom has always said that she wanted to die with her tennis shoes on, which I think exemplifies this perfectly. Which model of aging would you find preferable? I'm sure it's the dotted line!

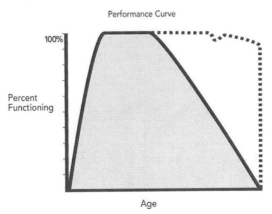

Performance Curve

100%

Percent
Functioning

Age

Let's also look at one of the most shocking, yet preventable changes that can happen as we age. In the sixty-year snapshot between our twentieth birthday and our eightieth birthday, the average person loses HALF of their leg strength if they are not purposefully trying to

We're constantly joking about the aches and pains of getting older. These stereotypes are part of the problem. When we assume something is inevitable, we stop trying to prevent it.

prevent it through exercise. Imagine what it would look like and feel like if you were to go through daily life with your current body weight, yet only half of your current leg strength. The math should work out to feel the same as if you doubled your body weight for your current leg strength. How would that feel trying to get through the day? You might need to shuffle when you walk. You would need to take breaks to sit down. You would be hunched over. Does this sound familiar, like some 85-year-olds you might encounter?

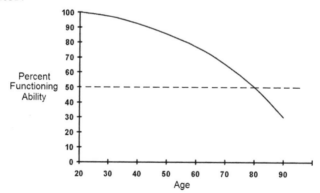

Look at this image comparing a cross section of the leg muscles and fat of a 74-year-old sedentary man with that of a 70-year-old triathlete.

74-year-old sedentary man

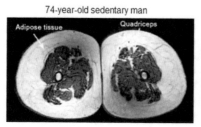

70-year-old triathlete

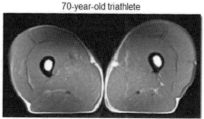

Quite a difference, huh? The significant muscle loss that happens to many individuals as they age is called *sarcopenia.* The great news is that the decline in muscle mass is to a large extent both *preventable* and *reversible*! No matter how late in life you start, the body will respond to exercise. The earlier we start, the better off we are.

A research study in 2018 at Ball State University found that individuals in their seventies who had been exercising most of their adult lives had muscles that were similar to that of 25-year-olds! There are research studies done with very frail, elderly people who began strength training at an advanced age with fantastic improvements and increases in strength through weight training exercise. In many cases, their results were significant enough to reduce or eliminate their need for walkers or canes.

For fitness professionals, working with older adults can shed a new perspective on some of the shallower, vanity-related goals that are commonly linked with fitness. Most older adults aren't exercising to show off their bodies on the beach; instead, examples of their goals might include being strong enough to travel to a grandchild's wedding or simply maintaining the ability to shower and dress oneself. These are not situations that many of us think about if we haven't been faced with caregiving in our lives.

For older adults who have experienced a decline in function to the extent that they need regular assistance with activities of daily living, it doesn't have to be a failure or a reason to give up hope for improvements in quality of life. Families and individuals can work with their caregivers to provide appropriate opportunities for movement and realistic goals for mobility.

What a wonderful, inspiring message it is that the muscles and the brain respond at any age, impacting mobility, agility, independence, metabolism, weight management, appearance at whatever weight you are, posture, back pain, and so much more! The "use it or lose it" principle extends to many of the physical ailments that we like to "blame" on age. Research tells us that *many of the changes that we commonly blame on age, are not due in total to the physiological aging process, but rather the gradual decline in activity—both physical and cognitive—that typically comes with aging.* It's something to think about! What type of 85-year-old do you want to be and are your current habits going to get you there? If your current lifestyle needs a little adjustment, that's ok. *It's NEVER TOO EARLY and it's NEVER TOO LATE!*

If lifestyle accounts for 70% of the differences in how people age and we want to age as healthfully as possible, it makes sense to look at examples of people who are doing it well. *The Blue Zones* by Dan Buettner tells us that there are three groups of people who have the greatest percentage of centenarians on the planet. A good portion of their elders live past the age of 100—quite a feat! These groups include Okinawans, Sardinians, and Seventh Day Adventists. If we want to increase our chances of living to 100, why not follow their example for lifestyle habits? What do they have in common?

- They don't smoke.
- They are active every day.
- They put family first.
- They maintain active social lives.
- They eat a diet high in fruits, vegetables, and whole grains.

Do these habits seem difficult or complicated? Of course not. Rather, they are probably things that many of us would like to do in theory if we aren't already, but in our busy or preoccupied lives, we don't prioritize because we don't think they will make that much of a difference. Perhaps it's time for a more serious effort, knowing what we have to gain. Time and again, we will encounter small changes that yield meaningful benefits!

There are also examples all around us of inspiring people who are challenging the stereotypes of aging. Check out Marc Middleton's website www.GrowingBolder.com for motivational profiles on older adults doing amazing things. From swimming champions, models on the catwalk, graceful ballerinas, and super strong yoga instructors, you are sure to be inspired!

NEVER TOO EARLY, NEVER TOO LATE: LET'S GET STARTED!

Regardless of your age or stage of life, isn't it time you took charge of your health and wellness if you haven't already? It doesn't matter where you are now or how great or small your ultimate aspirations are. You can get a stronger body, a sharper brain, and gain endless energy. Don't wait another day!

As you read along, look for the little sidebars that highlight thoughts and tips that are specifically more applicable for the NEVER TOO EARLY or the NEVER TOO LATE reader. I hope they resonate with you.

The NEVER TOO EARLY mindset proposes that if you start now, you'll stave off many of the ailments that might otherwise impact you as you age. The NEVER TOO LATE mindset proposes that regardless of your age or physical limitations, there are things you can do that will improve your health, mobility, and quality of life!

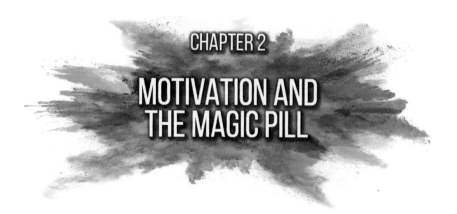

CHAPTER 2

MOTIVATION AND THE MAGIC PILL

ARE YOU FEELING motivated after understanding the urgency we are all facing? Capitalizing on that motivation will get us started laying the groundwork to achieve our strong body, sharp brain, and endless energy.

How to begin? We'll start with the *one thing*—the one action, one habit, one strategy that can have the greatest impact on all three of these goals at the same time. How efficient, right?! This *one thing* is so powerful in so many areas that I like to compare it to a magic pill. Imagine for a moment that there is indeed a pill with the following magical properties:

- Lowers your risk of heart disease, cancer, and diabetes.
- Increases your bone density, thereby decreasing your risk of osteoporosis.
- Conditions your heart and your lungs.
- **Strengthens your muscles (strong body).**
- Increases your metabolism.
- Improves your flexibility.
- Raises your HDL cholesterol (which is the good kind that you want to increase).
- Reduces back pain.

- Relieves stress and depression.
- Improves your blood pressure.
- Helps you sleep better.
- **Improves your mental skills (sharp brain).**
- Helps you lose weight.
- **Increases energy (endless energy).**
- Helps you maintain independence as you age.

Would you like this pill? Do I hear a resounding YES? It's hard to imagine someone not wanting this medication! Just a minute, though—there's a catch...

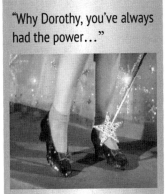

"Why Dorothy, you've always had the power…"

This pill is only dispensed in single daily doses, meaning you can't get a large bottle to last you all month. You must get each daily dose individually each day, and if taken as prescribed, the results are virtually guaranteed. (Take another look at the list of benefits noted to remind yourself of all that you have to gain if you take this pill.) The magical pharmacy that dispenses it is nearby, but in a pedestrian-only zone. It's about a half-mile away, meaning that you'll need to walk about ten minutes to get there and another ten minutes back.

Would you do it? Would you take twenty minutes out of your day to go get your daily dose if the benefits were virtually guaranteed? Hmmm...What's your answer? Still yes? What if I told you that the pill itself was completely worthless—just a placebo, and, in fact, *it was the daily twenty-minute walk that delivered the benefits, rather than the pill?*

Would you be surprised? A little disappointed? Would you say to yourself, "Aww, she's just talking about exercise!"?

The sad fact is that many of us have an easier time believing in a pill than in the capabilities of our own bodies. We are much more likely to put faith in the listed benefits of a medication than in the movement of our own bodies, over which we have control. The truth is that *exercise is the closest thing to a magic pill we will ever encounter*. Being active lowers your chance of developing over thirty diseases and troublesome medical conditions. This magic pill is not a chemical, herb, or any other product that you see on the shelves of a supplement store, yet people flock to supplements in their continual search for that one magic pill that will make a difference.

Here it is again: a magic pill does indeed exist, and it is called exercise. While this is not an exercise book, per se, if exercise is "the" main way for us to build a strong body AND a sharp brain AND endless energy, then exercise indeed deserves to be a major focus of this book! Let's take a third look at that list of benefits:

- Lowers your risk of heart disease, cancer, and diabetes.

- Increases your bone density, thereby decreasing your risk of osteoporosis.

- Conditions your heart and your lungs.

- **Strengthens your muscles (strong body).**

- Increases your metabolism.

- Improves your flexibility.

- Raises your HDL cholesterol (which is the good kind that you want to increase).

- Reduces back pain.

- Relieves stress and depression.

- Improves your blood pressure.

> **NEVER TOO EARLY**
> **Motivator**
>
> "Exercise helps reduce stress and lose weight? I could use some of that!"

> **NEVER TOO LATE**
> **Motivator**
>
> "Exercise helps my memory and helps relieve back pain? Sign me up!"

- Helps you sleep better.
- **Improves your mental skills (sharp brain).**
- Helps you lose weight.
- **Increases energy (endless energy).**
- Helps you maintain independence as you age.

And this is the short list! Check out "65 Reasons to Exercise" in the Appendix section and refer to it whenever you need a little motivation. There truly are at least sixty-five reasons to exercise. Exercise is arguably the single best thing you can do to invest in your health—delivering more benefits in more areas of your life than any other *single* action you can take. Taking this message to heart is the first step in gaining the benefits of fitness.

You can do many things that benefit your health in different ways, large and small—such as eating more fruits and vegetables, using sunscreen regularly, or reducing your salt or sugar intake. In fact, all of these changes will make a difference in some aspect of your health. However, none of those things, nor any other *single* thing you can do will have as many and as far-reaching health benefits in as many categories as E-X-E-R-C-I-S-E—moving your body!

WHAT ELSE?

Although we are kicking off with exercise, there are other key habits such as healthy eating, watching our weight, managing stress, getting enough sleep and much more that all tie together in reaching our trio of goals. We'll tuck away the other habits for now and address them later in the book. For now, we'll continue on with the magical pill called exercise. On the other hand, everything we are about to cover about the motivational side of fitness also applies to getting and staying motivated to stick with other healthy habits. Let's take a look.

IT'S A HARD PILL TO SWALLOW

If exercise really is the magic pill, why aren't we all exercising regularly? Why don't we have a huge fitness boom on our hands and a culture of physical activity? Despite the proven benefits of exercise, according to the 2018 Physical Activity Guidelines for Americans by the Department of Health and Human Services, 80% of American adults are not getting enough exercise to improve their health. Statistics also show that only 12-16% of Americans belong to a health club of some kind, and this speaks nothing of how many actually use their memberships! Our children aren't faring any better. Childhood obesity is on the rise. The effects are showing, literally, as we are a nation of growing girth.

THE WORLD WE LIVE IN MAKES IT TOUGH TO BE HEALTHY

No one said this was going to be easy. The American obsession with weight loss is at an all-time high. You can't open a magazine or turn on the TV without encountering yet another product or program guaranteed to help you lose weight. There are pills, potions, packaged foods, books, classes, websites, and gurus. Lots of people are making a lot of money, but are we getting anywhere?

Not likely.

America is as fat as ever . . . and getting fatter every year— meaning that the percentage of Americans in the "clinically obese" category has increased every year in the last twenty years. Let's look at an ongoing study by the Centers for Disease Control (CDC), which compares the percentage of each state's population who are considered clinically obese.

What could be causing this epidemic?

Let's begin with some commonplace habits today that would have Americans of an earlier era feeling puzzled.

Think about the prevalence and accessibility of packaged snack foods and fast food. When do we eat and what are we doing while we eat? In times gone past, we prepared meals at home and ate at the dinner table, while conversing with family or friends. Today, most meals for many people are consumed "on the run", in a restaurant, in the car, or in front of the TV. We are often numb while we shovel food mindlessly into our mouths.

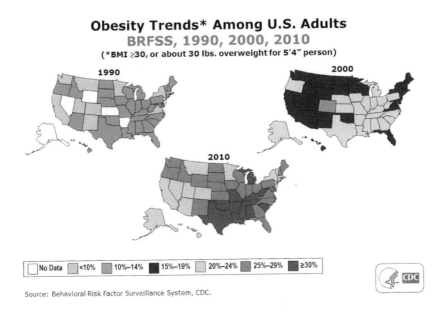

Obesity Trends* Among U.S. Adults
BRFSS, 1990, 2000, 2010
(*BMI ≥30, or about 30 lbs. overweight for 5'4" person)

No Data   <10%   10%–14%   15%–19%   20%–24%   25%–29%   ≥30%

Source: Behavioral Risk Factor Surveillance System, CDC.

Next, let's think about the "super-size syndrome". Envision the hamburger, salad, soda, or cookie of the 1950s. Now, think of the size of the hamburger, salad, soda, or cookie you'd purchase today. Chances are they are at least twice the size! Picture the sodas and flavored coffee beverages that are popular these days and the enormous sizes being sold. Many people are completely unaware how many calories per day they are *drinking*, on top of what they are eating. The more desensitized we become to these serving sizes, the more it becomes second nature to over-consume. Ask friends who come from a different culture and they will tell you that they have never seen a culture with eating habits quite like Americans. We eat and eat and then we eat some more! For all the talking we do about dieting, as a nation, we simply do not put our money where our mouths are.

Our activity habits for the most part, are no better. Generations ago, many Americans performed daily tasks that involved physical work—milking cows, plowing fields, or working in a factory. Today, most people live very sedentary lives. Oftentimes, we sit all day whether it's at home, at work, or in the car. Our culture and the very infrastructure of most towns and cities, especially in suburbia, rely heavily upon cars. Schools, shopping, and housing are no longer within walking distance in many communities. Many of us drive everywhere. Whether our destination is close or far, we hop in the car and go. Visiting our European and Asian counterparts, we would be stunned to witness their habit of walking and biking throughout their daily travels—physical activity is built into their day.

There is also the time factor. The pace of our lives has increased to the point that we expect instant results and instant gratification from everything that we do. There's an app for everything.

We are paying a dear price for our fast-paced lives and most of us don't even know it. We've slowly spoiled ourselves to the point that we avoid physical exertion at all costs. How many remote controls do you have in your household? We rush around in the morning to get in our cars and sit...we scurry quickly into work and sit...we circle and circle for the closest spot at the mall, and we make good use of elevators, escalators, and moving sidewalks at the airport. Many of us simply do not move our bodies unless absolutely necessary!

The CDC has compiled numerous health-related statistics. The health risks associated with our lifestyle—inactivity, poor nutrition, obesity, and smoking—now account for 51% of all deaths in the United States. Smoking is still the number one killer in America—35,000 deaths per year. Obesity is the second leading cause of preventable deaths in this country, with the last count at 26,000. How about the economic cost of obesity? One hundred billion dollars will be spent on the medical treatment of diseases caused by obesity, in addition to 65 billion dollars spent by consumers on the diet industry. Despite the money being spent, 95% of all diets fail!

THE INDIVIDUAL LAUNDRY LIST

Even though we live in a culture of inactivity, there still exists the opportunity to make our own decisions. What are the most common reasons why busy people don't exercise? See if any of the below sound familiar:

- I don't have time.
- I'm too tired.
- It's too boring.
- It's too hard.
- I don't need it.
- I'm too old.
- I don't have any equipment.
- It's too expensive.
- I don't need to lose weight.
- I've got a bad [back, knees, etc.].
- I don't like to sweat.
- It's not convenient.
- Nobody will go with me.
- I want to exercise in general, but I just never feel like exercising!

The list could go on and on. After a while, they all start to sound a little bit like "the dog ate my homework", don't they?

When we make excuses for something, it simply means that the motivator isn't strong enough. For example, if you were told you would receive $10,000 if you exercised for 20 minutes without fail three times per week for the next month, you'd find a way, wouldn't you? Conversely, if you were told that you had a life-threatening disease and that you would die if you didn't exercise for twenty minutes three times per week, every week, you'd also find time to do it, wouldn't you? Of course, you would. We find time or make time for those things that are most important to us, when we have what psychologists call a "personally compelling motivator". The thing that motivates us needs to be *personal* and it needs to be *compelling*. General, vague, and lukewarm reasons won't cut it. If you want to increase your chances of success in starting and sustaining a fledgling exercise routine, think about a reason that is personally compelling for you. You've just increased your chances of success!

You can also think about the many things you do that are such ingrained habits that they are "non-negotiable" daily tasks like showering, brushing your teeth, and dressing before you leave the house. Do you ever find yourself saying, "I just didn't have time"? No; you just do them. You don't complain, and you aren't looking for a pat on the back for getting them done. Why is exercise not in that category? What puts something into the non-negotiable, must-do category in your mind? Food for thought!

> **NEVER TOO EARLY**
> and
> **NEVER TOO LATE**
> **Real Reflections**
>
> "Yup, I see myself here. I've been making excuses. She makes some good points and these statistics are pretty convincing. I think I may need to change my ways!"

PRIORITY, HABIT, AND AN ACCURATE ASSESSMENT OF THE INVESTMENT NECESSARY

Priority and habit are the two markers of how we spend our time, with the caveat of an accurate assessment of what it takes to gain the benefits. If exercise is the single best way to get a strong body, a sharp brain, and endless energy, and if it's the single best way to improve our quality of life as we age, then we'd be crazy *not* to fit it in, wouldn't we? Well, that depends. The second half of the equation is an accurate assessment of how much exercise is necessary to receive the benefits. Many people feel overwhelmed because they think they need an extensive, time-consuming, complete lifestyle overhaul in order to gain any benefits. The good news—actually, the *great news* is that there are meaningful health improvements to be gained from even modest investments of time.

Take a close look at your reasons for not exercising regularly at this point if that's the case and be honest with yourself about the priorities in your life. If exercise is not a priority for you, hopefully it will become one by the time you finish reading this book. The first step is admitting where it falls on your priority list right now rather than rationalizing about your reasons for not exercising regularly. The reasons are real, but they are not insurmountable when exercise becomes a priority and when you realize that the amount of time needed to reap the benefits is less than you previously thought.

How does something (like exercise) magically move up the priority list? Let's start with the simple ratio of pros versus cons. The cons are your reasons why you can't exercise (time, inconvenience, etc.). These roadblocks certainly do exist and may overshadow the pros when you only have a few pros or reasons why you feel you should exercise. That is why we started off this chapter with the long list of benefits in our magic pill that *far* outweigh the challenges. The trick is to keep the benefits front and center in our minds and then address the challenges one by one.

Now that we have looked at all the reasons why you might not already have a strong exercise habit yet, let's move on to helping you move forward!

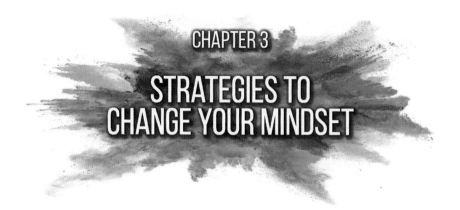

CHAPTER 3
STRATEGIES TO CHANGE YOUR MINDSET

H OW CAN WE get our minds on track to get our bodies moving and our expectations realistic? Having the right mindset is crucial to our success in fitting in exercise and other healthy habits. We are going to address the important business of getting rid of our mental baggage, fixing our mindset, and looking at our lifestyle commitments from a philosophical point of view that will keep us nourished for the long-term.

GETTING RID OF UNHEALTHY MINDSETS

Do you have an unhealthy mindset that is undermining your ability to feel good and be successful? The most common unhealthy mindsets are all-or-none thinking, pessimism, stereo-typing, and the mighty "quick fix."

All or None

Are you under the impression that it's full-throttle workout or bust? Many of us have heard the recommendations, read the "most effective exercises" for this, that, or the other...and feel obligated to do it a certain way or—well—*"It's not worth it...I might as well not do it at all."*

The truth is, there are many health benefits to be gained from even modest amounts of exercise. Have you ever skipped a workout when you thought it'd take too long? Think again. When you don't have time for your full routine, a shorter one will do. Too often, an all-or-none mentality robs us of the Holy Grail of exercise—consistency! Consistency is, in my opinion, the most important part of exercise. Would you believe that content is completely secondary? I have met with countless clients or potential clients throughout the years who want me to design the "perfect" exercise routine for them, but that doesn't mean they will do it, or that they will do it long enough to see the results. What good is the perfect routine if you can only stick to it for a few workouts or a few weeks? Wouldn't it be much better to start with a more modest, realistic exercise routine that you can build on?

> **NEVER TOO EARLY**
> **Menacing Mindsets**
>
> "I'm young and don't really have any health issues, so I don't really need to exercise. Who's got the time?"

One strategy that works very well is to have a full-fledged routine that you do when you have time, but you also have mini-exercise options for those busy days or weeks that serve a great purpose—*keeping you on track*. Ask yourself, "What's realistic today ... this week ... in general?" What's "good enough?" There are plenty of days on which good enough is truly good enough—a victory—a true success! Maybe your normal routine is 45 minutes of cardiovascular exercise and a 30-minute strength training routine. On a day when you are tired or pressed for time, wouldn't it be better to do a quick 20 minutes of cardiovascular exercise and then just one or two strength training exercises rather than doing nothing at all? Do not let perfectionism ruin your opportunity to get in some kind of workout.

Pessimism

Have you tried and failed before? Started and stopped a dozen times? Convinced yourself that you won't ever get fit or lose weight?

Often, we are our own worst enemy in mental mind games. Think of how you would speak to a close friend who was struggling to make a certain lifestyle change and kept faltering. Would you berate your friend? Or would you offer consolation and encouragement? Be a good friend to yourself and give yourself the gift of faith, understanding, and a second (or third or fourth) chance. You can do this! You are going to get the right information, cultivate the right expectations, and do something to improve your health! Do not give up!

Stereotypes and Self-Consciousness

Stereotypes in fitness are everywhere. Unfortunately, we are subjected to body-image baggage and athletic-ability baggage that can take the wind out of our sails with one look at the local health club's advertisements. Contrary to some images, already being fit, looking good in exercise clothes, or having been athletic or coordinated in high school are not prerequisites for exercising.

Fitness is for everybody ... but more importantly, it's for every *body*. Your body needs to move, and you shouldn't let anybody or anything make you feel too self-conscious or awkward, or old, or WHATEVER to do *something*. There is a huge variety of fitness options available beyond the glitzy, "everybody

> **NEVER TOO LATE**
> **Menacing Mindsets**
>
> "I'm too old and it's too late for me to gain any real benefit from exercise."

is staring at you" type of health club. Family-friendly clubs, older adult-friendly centers, and no-frills old-school "gyms" abound. Community centers have homey fitness centers and there is much you can do in the comfort of your own home.

For most of us, however, it's not a problem of other people stereotyping us. Rather, we've done it to ourselves! Are you guilty of categorizing *yourself* as a non-exerciser, a confirmed couch potato, or a lost cause? Have you declared that you don't *need* exercise because you don't need to lose weight? Even if exercise clothes and fitness centers are not for you, there is much you can do for your health. Research has shown that even a modest increase in physical activity can have a significant impact on your health. A mere 30 minutes or more of movement per day can decrease your risk of heart disease and a host of other ailments. The most important thing is finding something you enjoy and getting started!

The Quick Fix

The promise of the quick fix is certainly alluring, but unfortunately, it's short-lived and all your dreams of "body beautiful in 30 days" are dashed. Results are often promised in record time and when they don't happen, we end up demoralized and defeated until the next try. This can be a never-ending cycle of overly stringent "on" periods, followed by sheepish or decadent "off" periods.

The roller coaster doesn't do our bodies or minds any good and it certainly doesn't lead to the results we want. Unfortunately, what works just isn't quick. Are you ready to stop looking for a quick fix? Can you truly accept that it doesn't exist? Are you ready to negotiate how much you are willing to give (in terms of diet and exercise changes) and accept what your body (given your genetics) is willing to do with that level of change? Everyone is different, and your exercise and nutrition plan need to be realistic for your life—*your whole life*—in order to work. The best plan means nothing if you can't stick with it. Try making one small change, then another, then another. Make the behavior the goal, not the result. Things have a way of building on one another.

When you make a few changes, ask yourself, *"Can I see myself doing this forever?"* If so, keep it up and see if you're able to reach your goals with that level of lifestyle change. If the results aren't enough for your desires, ask yourself if you're willing to make a few more changes forever and see what results that brings. Slow and steady wins the race.

I have a Nike poster hanging in my exercise room that shows a woman sitting on a weight bench wiping her brow. The slogan under the photograph reads, "There is no finish line." It reminds me every day that this is not a race, that I'm in this for the long haul, and that I'm just enjoying the ride with no intention of stopping.

Did you see yourself in any of these menacing mindsets? It's hard to change your thinking overnight, but you can start replacing some of those ingrained messages and put yourself on the right track.

ACCEPTING OWNERSHIP AND ADMITTING PRIORITIES

Important versus Urgent

Once you realize that an exercise program doesn't have to take a lot of time to be valuable, it breaks down a lot of the excuses we have. If you're still stuck, you need to stop blaming other things for your stalled exercise habits in order to move forward. Accepting ownership means realizing that you are in control of your daily life and your decisions on how to spend your time. We all have twenty-four hours in a day, and it is up to us how we choose to spend them. Some people have more discretionary time than others, but when we are honest with ourselves, we know that time is not the real issue. Regardless of how busy you are, exercise is one thing you can't delegate. Nobody can exercise for you!

> **NEVER TOO EARLY Motivator**
>
> "No more excuses. I can find time and I can make time."

Think about your workouts from the point of view of "important" versus "urgent". By now, you probably believe that exercise is important. The problem is that each individual exercise session will never be urgent, which is why it's so easy to cancel. Keep in mind the notion that each workout is important from the standpoint of keeping you on track, in addition to the actual benefits of the exercise session.

Finding Time versus Making Time

Finding time and making time are both great tools for accepting ownership and admitting your priorities. What's the difference between the two?

Finding time means keeping your eye out for little snippets of time that can make a big difference. How about getting up early one day a week, carving out a midday chunk once a week, and committing to one exercise session every weekend? If that sounds appealing, it's one example of how you could exercise three times per week without undue changes on any *one* part of your schedule.

Making time means examining your priorities and the things that are using up your time right now. Are there things that are taking up chunks of time that are not very fulfilling or valuable that you might want to cut out in order for you to make room for exercise? Are there things you could delegate?

Know Thyself—Preferences and Personality

Are you someone who likes to have alone time when you exercise or do you crave a fun, social atmosphere? That might mean the difference between joining an exercise class versus taking walks on your own. Do you prefer variety and become bored easily or are you most successful when you have a structured, predictable workout that you don't have to think about? When is your energy level highest? Are you an early morning person or a night owl? Do you like to chop things up into small, manageable bites, or "get it all over with"? Do you become overwhelmed easily, or do you prefer to dive into new things? All of these factors will impact your success level. Don't fool yourself. Your fitness plan must fit your preferences and your personality to be successful.

Anticipate and Strategize around Obstacles

We all have obstacles to changing our schedule, but most aren't insurmountable; they just require thoughtful strategizing and a commitment to stay the course despite a little drifting. No new habit is born overnight. And most obstacles do not appear overnight. Since most of your obstacles are indeed predictable, you can anticipate them and plan for how you will handle them. And you need practice handling them. Many fitness efforts fail because the perfect scenario is the only situation you've planned for. Recall the section on all-or-none thinking. This is where it is applied. Be sure that you develop back-up plans and a "good enough" mindset for days when you need to stay on track but can't do your normal routine.

Find a Common Thread to Stay on Track

One of the most valuable factors that can contribute to your success, especially during the fragile beginning period, is a common thread that strings the weeks together to become months and then years of a sensible approach and a healthy lifestyle. Remember, you're just living your life, in a healthier way, but slow and steady. You are not on a crash course to fitness and then you're done. Your common thread could be a personal trainer that you see at regular intervals (exactly how often may be determined by your budget), or a wellness coach. It could be an exercise class if you've developed friendships and camaraderie there, or a neighbor or family member who is just as committed to this as you.

Some of us have an old exercise buddy with whom we have a history of talking each other out of exercising or who cancels frequently. This person is not your common thread. Your common thread helps you stay the course over time. Your fitness level is defined by what your habits are at the time. You can't save it up. Keep up the habits and you keep that level of fitness; keep that level of health and wellness!

The "Click" Factor

You know when something just goes "click" in your brain? For whatever reason, you've mentally turned a corner and you're ready to do things differently. It makes sense and you feel the energy and the commitment. You get it and there's no going back. The click may happen when you suddenly encounter a really compelling motivator to make a certain change. Sometimes it's a catastrophic event—a parent having a heart attack at a young age, a diagnosis of an illness like diabetes. Sometimes it's a doctor's appointment where the doctor tells you that "if you continue on this path..."

The click could happen reading this book, it could happen when you see an old friend who has lost fifty pounds and is feeling on top of the world. The click sometimes comes a little more gradually before you know it happened. You may not know you have it until you

NEVER TOO LATE Motivator

"I am not too old and it is not too late!"

have the flu and it occurs to you that you miss working out and can't wait to get back to the gym. You might be standing at the kitchen sink mentally going through your day, and you realize getting in a workout is the first thing on your mind. You can't necessarily predict when it's going to happen, but you can continue to expose yourself to the positive messages and work towards your new healthy habits. Envision yourself already there and move toward it.

Practical Keys to Making It Work

You're still in planning mode, and it's time to take a quick look at a few considerations that really make a difference.

- Fun – Taking a walk can be relaxing alone time. Taking an exercise class can be great social time. Bike riding with family members can be a bonding time. Whatever it is . . . if it's not something you enjoy, it's no wonder you're not sticking to it. It doesn't have to be conventional; just move your body and have fun.

- The matter-of-fact approach – This may seem contradictory to the previous idea of making sure it's fun. Different things work for different people. If you look through the lens of "chores", we all have tasks that we don't particularly enjoy but are non-negotiable, such as cleaning the bathroom, or paying bills, or taking medicine. We may look for ways to keep it short and just check it off the list.

- Convenience – Look for what makes sense within your normal daily routine and travels. You may discover an exercise option close to work or home.

- Plan it into your day – Make your fitness routine just as much of a "given" as anything else on your to-do list. Plan specific days and times for your workouts.

- Flexibility and a back-up plan – Remember, a back-up plan and small ways to do "something" when you can't do your normal routine is key to keeping yourself active and on track. Travel, a sick family member, and deadlines at work can spell trouble unless you've already figured out what you'll do when obstacles arise.

- Put it on your appointment calendar and treat it like any other appointment.

- Once it's on your calendar, protect its place on the schedule. This goes back to the notion that fitness is important, but each individual exercise session is not urgent. When you plan to include exercise in your day, it must be with a fair amount of conviction. Don't be "too quick" to give up that spot to a competing demand. Use your back-up plan when necessary but be cautious when it begins to look like it's happening all the time.

Supportive Philosophical Musings—It's All in the Attitude

Staying in the right mindset is important. Our thoughts cause our feelings. Therefore, what you fill your brain with determines your mindset. Reading motivational books and articles, watching motivational programs, and seeking out positive role models all make a difference. How about what you say to yourself? Try to pay attention to your internal dialogue—the little voice that talks to you inside your head all day. Is it a positive voice or a negative voice? Attitude makes a big difference! Take a look at my free-flowing thoughts on fitness and a healthy outlook on personal wellness. I wrote it quite a few years ago, but it still holds true today.

Cathy's Fitness Philosophy

I believe that personal wellness is dynamic—that it is a journey, not a destination. It's figuring out what fits into your life at any given point— balancing the job of caring for the body you've been given with enjoying the life you've been given. I sometimes think that too many people put off feeling good about themselves until "after"-after they lose ten pounds, after they fit into a certain pair of jeans, after they stay on the "XYZ" diet successfully for "x" number of weeks. I believe in feeling good and accepting your body now, and then gradually taking small steps that don't cost much but will add up in the long run. Most people who go that route find that the small successes motivate them to add more and bigger changes down the road. I always encourage clients to only make changes that they can see themselves still doing a year from now. Many people aren't ready for that approach, though. After all, it goes against our natural tendency to seek the short-term payoff. We live in a society of immediate gratification and promises of quick fixes and instant results. But how many more times do you want to start, fall off, and then re-start that stringent eating and exercise routine, each time re-calculating the date by which you'll see a certain result if you start again "now"? Sadly enough, those poorly patched-together weeks fly by until it is a year later and you are in the same place as when you started.

Why not take a different approach? Start with the long-term goal in mind from the beginning. What changes and habits can you incorporate into your life that you can see yourself doing—open-ended— just because you've decided "that's the way you live your life now"? Something has to click inside you to be ready. And when you're ready, you need support and continuity—a common thread of some kind that will help you stay the course through the weeks and months until you've found the part within you that will keep it going on your own. I believe in the power of taking charge of your life— reflecting on what you want your life to be and then making intentional choices to help that goal to materialize. I believe in focusing on the habits and actions that build health, rather than focusing on the result. If you focus on enjoying today and enjoying the journey, you will see the results along the way.

My challenge to you is to establish an attitude for success. Internalize these thoughts:

- This is a long-term process.
- It's a choice, a priority, and a lifestyle.
- You're ready to accept that there are no quick fixes.
- You're done with extremes.
- It's about forever.
- There is no finish line.
- There is no hurry to arrive. There is no train to catch.
- It's about making small changes little by little that you have no intention of ever stopping.
- You are building good health and fitness from the inside out.
- Strive for consistency, not perfection.

- Focus on the actions, not the outcomes.
- You will be giving yourself the gift of doing something good for yourself.
- Those small, good choices will slowly add up.
- Time will pass and you will still be doing those things.
- Small health changes lead to bigger health changes.
- The results will come. Do they really have to come within a preconceived time frame in order to have been worthwhile?
- Be positive, be easy on yourself, and treat yourself as a friend.
- Take one day and one week at a time.
- You are positive, flexible, and resilient. Let it shine through!
- Avoid complaining about how you look (especially if you are a woman with daughters) and about aches and pains. Accept who and where you are now and move forward.
- Change your environment to set yourself up to succeed! Do not rely on "willpower" while you are unequipped with the things you need to succeed amidst a sea of temptations.
- Fight the good fight. Make a good faith effort to practice habits that are as healthy as you're willing to sustain and then accept the outcome as what's meant to be.
- Stop comparing yourself to neighbors, friends, celebrities, or the people featured on advertisements. Your body and your response to eating and exercise changes are unique to you.

With a positive mindset as our new base, let's move on to the next step and decide what *actions* to take!

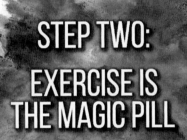

STEP TWO:

EXERCISE IS
THE MAGIC PILL

CHAPTER 4
EXERCISE BASICS AND THE NEVER TOO EARLY AND NEVER TOO LATE PHILOSOPHY

W E'VE ESTABLISHED THAT physical exercise is the single best strategy for all three of our goals of having a strong body, a sharp brain, and endless energy. Those who aren't thrilled at the prospect of exercise will be pleased to know that there are benefits from simply moving more without changing into exercise clothes or doing a specific regimen.

NEVER TOO EARLY

For many years, I have been using the phrase "the bare minimum" to describe an exercise attitude that many people can relate to. I first started using this terminology when I was working in corporate wellness and one day someone came to meet with me and said, "Look, I know I need to exercise. I don't have time to do much. I don't want to do much. Can you just give me the bare minimum I need to get by, so that I can feel good that I'm finally taking care of this major 'should' in my life?"

Many busy people avoid consulting with fitness professionals because they're too embarrassed to admit to someone—whose life revolves around fitness—that they don't really like it very much. They worry that they'll end up with a time-consuming, unrealistic exercise plan plus a generous helping of even more guilt. All they really want is a modest program, so they can check it off their list and be able to say to themselves, "Yes, I'm addressing this area of my life." Their goals and approach are valid and worthwhile. A minimalist exercise approach is both possible and valuable!

The exercise strategies and sample recommendations in this book that are labeled "*NEVER TOO EARLY*" are not only about age. They are geared towards those with a higher physical capacity. There will certainly be some individuals who are well into their later years who are able to use the "*NEVER TOO EARLY*" exercise routines, likely due to a consistent exercise history and impressive health and mobility. Fantastic!

NEVER TOO LATE

In addition to working in corporate wellness, I also spent many years working in a senior living setting. Some older adults are intimidated with exercise because it doesn't fit how they see themselves. They might not own any athletic clothing and assume all exercise is strenuous and designed for younger, more nimble bodies. Nothing is farther from the truth. There are meaningful, valuable exercise routines that can be designed for anyone, at any age, with any health conditions, and with any mobility challenges. There are fitness professionals who specialize in exercise recommendations and modalities that are especially designed for older adults to give them the benefits they need and deserve.

The exercise strategies and sample recommendations in this book that are labeled "NEVER TOO LATE" are also not only about age. A younger individual, who has dealt with health or mobility setbacks or otherwise needs a more conservative and gentle exercise strategy will be well-suited for the "NEVER TOO LATE" exercise routines.

Whether you identify with *NEVER TOO EARLY* or *NEVER TOO LATE*, one of my favorite phrases is:

> "More may be better than less, but some is better than none."

You don't have to be interested in doing a lot in order to benefit from exercise. Remember, with exercise, there are meaningful gains from even modest investments of time.

EXERCISE HOW-TO

There is an exercise strategy that can work for everyone. If you are a true skeptic and/or want to do as little as possible, you'll be pleased to know that there is a level called *"Just MOVE"*—as simple as that.

When you think about starting an exercise program, you may not know what type of benefits you can gain from different kinds of exercise. A new client might complain to me, "I've been doing abdominal work every day, and I can't seem to get rid of the fat on my stomach!" Unfortunately, that's no surprise. Exercises that target the abdominal *muscles* do nothing for the *fat lying on top of the abdominal muscles*. Abdominal strengthening exercises will help improve the overall appearance of your abdominal region, but they do so by making the stomach muscles firmer.

Decreasing the fat lying on top of the abdominal muscles is only possible when you burn more calories than you consume with some help from Mother Nature. Some of us genetically store more fat in the abdominal region, others in the hip and thigh region. Wherever your trouble spot is, it's stubborn for a reason!

So how do you develop the right expectations and select the right kind of exercise for you? Let's start with the three categories of exercise that benefit *everyone*. In a perfect world, you'd be doing "something" from each of these three categories but using our "some is better than none" philosophy, choose what most interests you and perhaps it will grow to more in the future.

1. Cardiovascular/Aerobic Exercise

2. Strength Training

3. Flexibility/Stretching

Let's take a closer look at each of these three important areas by devoting a chapter to each one. Next, we'll build on that knowledge.

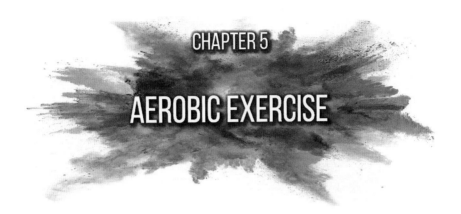

CHAPTER 5

AEROBIC EXERCISE

CARDIOVASCULAR ENDURANCE AND aerobic endurance are interchangeable terms, thought by many people to be the most important component of fitness. Whichever term you use, it's defined as the strength and efficiency of your heart, lungs, and blood vessels. Your well-conditioned heart and blood vessels go a long way in the prevention of heart disease and in your capacity to comfortably participate in a variety of activities in your day-to-day life. Your aerobic fitness level will determine whether you get winded if you must go up a flight of stairs or hurry to catch up to someone.

There's only one way to improve cardiovascular endurance and that is through aerobic exercise, which involves moving large muscle groups at a subjectively measured "somewhat hard" level for an extended period of time, usually around 20 minutes or more. Examples include walking, jogging, biking, swimming, using an elliptical machine, or aerobic dance classes.

Aerobic means "with oxygen", so for an activity to qualify, you must be able to continue to breathe and move without needing to stop to catch your breath. Whether an activity is considered aerobic for you depends on your fitness level. You might be able to sustain continuous breathing while brisk walking, but not while jogging; or maybe you can sustain a slow jog, but not a fast jog.

Each person needs to moderate their intensity so that it feels somewhat hard, but sustainable for 20 minutes or more. If 20 minutes of any movement is too much, you can start with even five minutes and build up from there.

The benefits of aerobic exercise are far-reaching, making it incredibly valuable for anyone. The benefits don't stop with improving the efficiency of your heart and lungs. The list goes on and on! You can also improve your muscular endurance and brain fitness, decrease your risk of heart disease, diabetes, certain cancers, and a host of other diseases and ailments. And because you burn so many calories per minute during aerobic exercise, it helps with weight loss and/or weight maintenance. If the activity is weight bearing (meaning that you're standing up during it), it improves bone density, which decreases your risk of osteoporosis. Quite a list, huh?

NEVER TOO EARLY Examples

Jogging/running
Brisk walking
Standing elliptical
Swimming
Deep water running
Cycling
Aerobic classes (i.e. Zumba, dance aerobics, etc.)

NEVER TOO LATE Examples

Walking
Seated elliptical
Recumbent cycle
"NuStep" machine
Water walking
Deep water running
Swimming
*Aquatic exercise feels great for joints!

There are plenty of other modes of aerobic exercise and as you can see, plenty of overlap in the "NEVER TOO EARLY" and "NEVER TOO LATE." Choose what you enjoy and what feels good for your body.

HOW OFTEN, HOW HARD, AND HOW LONG?

Remember that in order to be considered aerobic, the exercise needs to use large muscle groups and elevate your heart rate for an extended period of time. The traditional criteria that need to be met in order to gain the benefits of aerobic exercise have been outlined by the American College of Sports Medicine (www.acsm.org).

1. Frequency: typically, 3–5 times per week
2. Intensity: "somewhat hard" to "hard"
3. Duration: typically, 20–60 minutes

Let's look at each criterion in more detail:

Frequency — "How often?"

It's recommended that you do some form of aerobic exercise at least three times per week to give your body a frequent enough stimulus to force it to adapt. The fitness principles of overload and overcompensation are at work when you place more of a demand on your body than what it is used to, causing your body to adapt so it can handle those same demands in the future. These principles really kick in with a frequency of three times per week. If you exercise less than three times per week, your body may be thinking, "Why adapt when I'm not asked to work this hard very often?"

What about doing aerobic exercise more than three times per week? It is common to do aerobic exercise as little as three times per week or up to five or even seven days per week. Seven days per week is unnecessary—one day of rest is always a good idea, especially for your joints, so you don't risk "overtraining".

If you are doing more and more exercise and seeing less results, your body may be telling you it needs a break. However, some people really enjoy their exercise time and want to do it almost every

NEVER TOO EARLY
and
NEVER TOO LATE
Frequency

I don't recommend less than three times per week for anyone. Give your body the frequent enough stimulus to get the benefits!

Even six days a week isn't too much for "NEVER TOO LATE" as long as the intensity is not too high and there is no pain.

day. If you are careful to mix in at least several days a week of low intensity, easy-on-the-joints activities (like walking), you may be able to exercise seven days a week without a problem. Four or five days a week is very common for those who really enjoy their routine. Obviously, the more days per week you exercise, the more calories you will burn and the higher your cardiovascular conditioning. General health conditioning can be achieved with just three days per week while those who are trying to lose weight will probably find that they need 5–6 days per week in order to really impact their weight loss results.

"How hard?" — Intensity

There are many ways to measure or estimate intensity of aerobic exercise. Remember that the goal for aerobic exercise is to work at an intensity that you can sustain for twenty minutes or more. Some individuals might start with less than twenty minutes and that's okay. Several factors determine whether you should measure your intensity more accurately or use a less-exact method of estimation. Let's look at the different methods in order of simplest to most complex.

1. The "Talk Test"
You should feel like you can talk while you are exercising, but you should prefer not to talk very much! If you feel like you can't talk at all, your intensity is probably too high. If you feel like you could tell your life story while exercising, your intensity is probably not high enough!

NEVER TOO EARLY Intensity

If you feel like pushing yourself, feel free to go up to an RPE of "hard". You could also try interspersing high intensity intervals for added interest.

NEVER TOO LATE Intensity

It shouldn't feel like a walk in the park, but you will probably want to stay on the conservative side. Shoot for an RPE of "somewhat hard" at the highest.

If you are feeling nauseous or over extended, you are probably overdoing it. There's no need for that. Listen to your body and ease up. There are still benefits from a moderate intensity level.

2. "Rate of Perceived Exertion" (RPE)

There is a scale that rates your subjective perception of how hard you are exercising from very light to light to somewhat hard to hard to very hard. General advice is that the exercise should feel "somewhat hard" for beginners. For more advanced exercisers, "hard" is okay, too. If exercise feels "light" or "very hard", it means your heart is probably beating too fast or too slow for an aerobic workout.

3. Target Heart Rate

Counting your heart rate or using a heart rate monitor is a common method of assessing your aerobic exercise intensity, especially in organized, class settings. For most people who have more casual goals, I have found the talk test or the rate of perceived exertion to be sufficient. If you are working with a fitness professional who would like to more closely monitor your intensity, or if you have special concerns, such as cardiac rehabilitation, you will likely be given a more specific target heart rate range to work within and will be prompted to measure your heart rate frequently during exercise.

"How long?" — Duration

How long does your aerobic workout need to be? We've already established that 20 minutes is the traditional minimal recommendation for cardiovascular benefits. However, research now shows that there is much to be gained from shorter amounts of exercise, especially compared to doing nothing.

The 20-minute recommendation is based primarily on improving cardiovascular fitness and heart health. If you are interested in losing weight, however, you will probably find that 20 minutes isn't quite enough. More committed and enthusiastic individuals and those who want to lose weight often

NEVER TOO EARLY Duration

You will probably feel as though 20-30 minutes is quite enough. If the intensity is low, you may enjoy extending to 40 minutes or so.

NEVER TOO LATE Duration

Trust your body and stop when you are fatigued.

spend 30, 40, or even 60 minutes doing their aerobic workout. It is definitely something you need to build up to.

Also, it should make sense that duration and intensity are closely linked. If you have a long workout, you will probably lower your intensity a bit. Conversely, for shorter workouts, you may find that you can push yourself a little...or not! Either way is fine. In general, it is a great idea to vary the duration of your aerobic workouts. Maybe you'll decide to do several 20-minute higher intensity workouts during the week and use the weekend to try to get in a longer one. Regardless, any amount of time is fantastic!

VARIATION

It is a good idea to vary the kind of aerobic exercise that you do. For instance, I wouldn't recommend that you always use an elliptical machine or only jog. It is good to vary the method of exercise so that you are not stressing the same muscles and joints the same way with each workout. This will help prevent overuse injuries. It is especially unwise to do high impact exercises, such as running, all the time, as this puts a lot of stress on your joints.

Also, from a fitness improvement standpoint, you want to keep your body guessing. If you always do the same workout the same way, your body becomes very efficient at it and you won't reap as many benefits as if you occasionally switched things around. There's also something called "Interval Training" where you alternate short spurts of a higher intensity level with longer periods of lower intensity. If this appeals to you, give it a try! There is no need to overthink the exact ratio of higher to lower intensity. Your body will likely tell you!

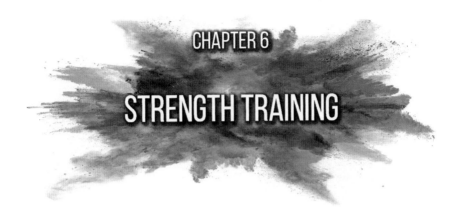

CHAPTER 6

STRENGTH TRAINING

MUSCULAR STRENGTH IS the maximal amount of force that your muscles can generate in one effort (Can you lift this heavy box or not?) Muscular endurance is the ability of your muscles to exert a smaller level of force over an extended period. (How far can you carry this medium-sized box before you need to set it down?)

The primary way to improve muscular strength is through some type of strength training routine. This can be in the form of weight training with dumbbells, weight machines, elastic tubing, or body weight exercises.

Strength training targets each muscle group, one by one, with the intention of fatiguing that muscle by applying resistance against it while the muscle contracts. The resistance must be challenging in order to gain significant benefits—you can't just go through the motions. Muscles grow and adapt when they are overloaded. If the resistance is not challenging, you will not grow stronger. The number one mistake many people make is lifting weights that are too light and wondering why they aren't seeing any changes. The second biggest mistake people make is lifting weights that are too heavy and hurting themselves. I'll explain how to get *just* the right weight for you.

The benefits of strength training are extensive and often not appreciated, which is why I refer to it as your secret weapon for a strong body, sharp brain, and endless energy! In addition to developing stronger, firmer muscles, you will also increase your metabolic rate to allow you to burn more calories all day long—at rest, during exercise, and all throughout the day.

NEVER TOO EARLY
Strength Training

Do it, do it, do it! Rack up those benefits that will serve you for years to come!

NEVER TOO LATE
Strength Training

Don't be intimidated! It's one of the BEST things for you, especially for prevention of osteoporosis and reducing your fall risk!

The terms resistance training, weight training, and strength training are interchangeable. Whatever you call it, and whatever type of equipment you use—the act of using muscular force against a resistance—forces your muscles to respond and adapt.

Almost any kind of exercise will have a positive impact on your muscles, but resistance training is the most powerful way to do so. Women have a significant opportunity to benefit from building their muscles, because they naturally have a smaller percentage of muscle on their bodies than men. Young or old, thin or heavy— weight training equals increased metabolism, a firmer looking body, better blood sugar regulation, and more stable joints. You can't afford *not* to do some form of resistance training!

If it's so great, why do so many people shy away from resistance training? Do you see yourself in any of these scenarios?

- Many people stick with what they know—which is usually limited to aerobic exercise.

- Some people think that if their primary objective is to lose weight, they should focus only on aerobic exercise and save weight training until "after" they lose weight (which never comes).

- Some women are put off by the misconception that lifting weights is a masculine thing.

- Some men are put off by the misconception that lifting weights is a "muscle head thing".
- Some women are worried that they'll build unsightly bulky muscles.
- Some people are embarrassed that they don't know how to use the machines and don't want to look silly or injure themselves.

Once you understand the enormous benefits and see that it doesn't have to be intimidating, you will open up a whole new world of exercise!

You can expect the following fantastic benefits when you embark on a weight-training program:

- Increased Round-the-Clock Metabolism
- A Firmer-Looking Body
- A Stronger You
- Help with Blood Sugar Regulation
- Stronger Bones
- Fall Risk Reduction
- Increased Joint Stability

Increased Round-the-Clock Metabolism

When you think of burning calories, do you automatically think of exercise? Think again! Even when you are just sitting around, doing nothing, your body is burning calories. In fact, your resting metabolic rate (the number of calories your body burns twenty-four hours a day, even at rest) typically contributes 60–75% of the total number of calories you burn in a day. In a rough estimate, while at rest, many people burn approximately one calorie per minute, or sixty calories per hour.

Muscle is the most important factor that determines whether you burn slightly more or less than the one calorie per minute estimate, making weight training possibly *the single best investment* you can make in increasing your resting metabolic rate. And when you impact your resting metabolic rate, you impact total calories in a big way.

If you think of your metabolism as a fire, then imagine the muscle cell as the furnace. Your muscle cell is "the" calorie-burning machine in your body. Weight training increases the size and efficiency of your muscle cells, giving you a larger and stronger furnace. Therefore, the more muscle you have, the more calories you burn all throughout the day—at rest, while going about the business of your day, and during exercise.

Do you burn many calories during your weight-training workout itself? Well, not really . . . especially when compared to aerobic exercise for the same amount of time. The important thing to keep in mind is that the benefits of weight training are not measured in a single workout. Rather, weight training is an investment in total calories that you burn the other 23 hours of the day. This information might explain why men usually have an advantage when it comes to metabolism. Some women might complain; "He can eat anything without gaining weight!"

It's a valid scenario. Pound for pound, when comparing a man and a woman of the same weight, the man will typically have substantially more muscle on his body. It gives women all the more reason to do as much as they can to increase their muscle mass. Since most women are starting with smaller muscles, they sometimes see the greatest gains when they begin a strength-training program. This is also true for men who have never tried it and many older adults. If you are not doing some form of weight training, you are missing a valuable opportunity to impact your metabolism.

A Firmer-Looking Body

Muscle provides the shape and contour of our body. Aerobic exercise is wonderful and will always be wonderful. But, if you are doing only aerobic exercise, you are missing the opportunity to change the shape of your body. When you lose weight through diet and aerobic exercise alone, you may lose weight, but you may also end up with simply a smaller version of your current body shape.

A Stronger You

We need muscular strength a lot more than we think to get through our daily activities, especially as we age. "Use it or lose it" definitely applies here. No matter your daily schedule of physical requirements, strong muscles will serve you well and stave off aches and pains. Muscles that are used to working hard respond to difficulties by rebuilding even stronger for next time. Strong leg muscles are the best way to improve balance, which is very important to prevent falls as we age.

Help with Blood Sugar Regulation

Working muscles need fuel, and when muscles spend a lot of time working, they absorb fuel really well. Muscle cells need to extract energy (glucose) from the bloodstream and they need to be receptive to the hormone insulin to do so. An inactive muscle may have a hard time letting insulin do its job of escorting glucose to the muscle cells. The glucose is available in the bloodstream, but it can't get into the muscle where it is needed. The pancreas compensates by secreting even more insulin into the bloodstream, trying to get the muscles to respond.

Does increased insulin and increased blood sugar floating aimlessly around the bloodstream make you think of something? (You guessed right if you're thinking about a breeding ground for diabetes.) To put "icing on the cake", there is one location that will eagerly accept excess blood sugar and make good use of high insulin levels: your fat cells. Strong muscles and regular exercise can change your body's chemistry and hormones and help your muscle cells absorb blood sugar before the fat cells can get to it. Any takers?

Stronger Bones

Strength training exercise is one of the best ways to build stronger bones and lower your risk of osteoporosis. Every time you work your muscles against a resistance, you are putting stress (the good kind) on your bones as well. This helps increase your bone density, which is often very desirable for women, especially as they age. As we age, hormonal changes often cause our bones to become less dense and therefore at higher risk of breaking, should we experience a fall. Safeguard your bones as best as you can with a regular strength training program!

Fall Risk Reduction

The best way to reduce your risk of falling is to have strong legs. You achieve this by having a consistent strength training routine so that you can walk sure-footedly in your day-to-day life. More on this later!

Increased Joint Stability

When you think of the location of a muscle, picture which joint it crosses. After all, the purpose of each muscle is to create movement. Every muscle in your body must cross one or more joints to create movement. The biceps cross the elbow joint and the quadriceps cross the knee joint. When the muscle is strong, it encases the joint in a more stable way and reduces your risk of joint injury. The strong muscle is better equipped to withstand an unexpected force placed on a joint when you stumble or have an accident. So, "having bad knees" for example, is not a good reason to avoid leg exercises; it's a reason to do them (carefully designed and performed correctly, of course)!

The Take-home Message

Have you figured out the message yet? You need to be doing some form of resistance training exercise. It doesn't have to be fancy. It doesn't have to be extensive. Whether you're young, old, injury-plagued, or short on time, there is a strength-training routine that can work for you. Whether it's a fitness center routine, a 10-minute home program with a few sets of dumbbells and elastic tubing, or bicep curls with soup cans, there is so much to be gained.

HOW TO CREATE YOUR WEIGHT TRAINING ROUTINE

Just as with aerobic exercise, you can do a short, minimalist routine, or a more comprehensive one, depending on your interest level and time. For a *comprehensive* resistance training routine, you'll want to do one or more exercises for each of the following major muscle groups. Remember, you may very well decide to only train a few of these muscle groups for now. You can tuck this information away for when you are ready for more.

Upper Body
- Shoulders
- Chest
- Back
- Biceps (front of the arm)
- Triceps (back of the arm)
- Abdominals (stomach area)

Lower Body
- Quadriceps (front of the thigh)
- Hamstrings (back of the thigh)
- Gluteus Maximus (rear end)
- Hip Abductors
- Inner Thigh/Adductors

Professional Instruction

One of the best ways to gain peace of mind that you are performing the right exercises for you and that you are performing them correctly, is to consult with a certified fitness professional. Make your goals clear as you look for the right person to work with. Quite often, you can find free or inexpensive access to a qualified fitness professional where you

Custom Strength Training Exercise Plans for
NEVER TOO EARLY
AND
NEVER TOO LATE

"How do these strength training exercise principles specifically apply to my situation?"

"Oh, that is coming in the next section? Thanks!"

live or work, or through a nearby fitness center. It can be a worthwhile investment to hire a personal fitness instructor to help you set up your program in the beginning if you plan to do your workout at home. They can then do periodic check-ins to adjust the program as needed and keep you motivated. It's a common misconception that working with a personal fitness trainer means having to pay someone to work with you for every workout. Consider setting a budget for this valuable investment on a periodic basis if you don't have other access. Your health is worth it!

Muscles That Work Together

When moving your body, very seldom does one muscle work alone. Most of the time, several muscle groups work together to cause movement, both in exercise and in real life. For instance, getting up out of a chair requires your hip and knee joints to move, thus requiring both your quadriceps along the front of your thighs and your gluteus maximus on your rear end to work together. Push-ups cause movement in your shoulder and elbow joints. Therefore, even though you think of push-ups as a chest exercise, they also work the triceps along the back of the arms. What does this mean for your exercise routine? Quite simply, that you can make good use of combination exercises that work several muscle groups together.

Tips for Sequencing Your Routine

In general, it is a good idea to work your large muscle groups before the smaller muscle groups that assist them. For instance, the triceps are involved in many chest exercises. If you work your triceps before your chest, you'll end up with arms that feel like spaghetti while you're trying to work your chest. The same rule applies for back and biceps. The biceps assist with your back exercises; therefore, it is better to work your back and chest first and your biceps and triceps after that.

Weight Training Lingo and Important Info

You'll feel a lot more comfortable with your exercise routine if you know the lingo and the background information for setting up a sound program. Here are a few terms and principles to know and understand:

Repetitions
"Reps" means repetitions, i.e. the number of times you perform an exercise before stopping. The traditional range for general conditioning is 8–15 repetitions of an exercise. Perform each repetition carefully and purposefully—typically a little faster on the first part (contraction) and a bit slower when you are returning to your starting position. You can pace yourself by counting "one... two..." on the way up (or whenever the muscle is contracting) and "one... two... three... four..." on the way back down (or when the muscle is elongating again).

How Many Reps Should I Do?
It should make sense that the heavier the weight is, the less repetitions you can do. And conversely, the lighter the weight, the more repetitions you can do. Twelve repetitions are the classic prescription for general conditioning, but it's common to perform anywhere between 8–15 repetitions. Research presented by the American College of Sports Medicine indicates similar strength and endurance benefits when you reach muscular fatigue anywhere within 8–15 repetitions. The most important factor is that you do indeed reach fatigue when you stop, at whatever number it happens to be within the 8–15 repetition range. The only difference within that range, according to the research, has to do with bone density. Research shows superior improvements in bone density when you use heavier weights and reach fatigue within the lower (8–10) repetitions range as opposed to using lighter weights and reaching fatigue within the higher (14–15) repetition range—great for reducing your risk of osteoporosis.

Select the Weight that Causes You to Reach Fatigue with this Range of Repetitions

The next important step is to select the weight that will cause you to **reach fatigue** within 8–15 repetitions. **This is perhaps the most important piece of information about effective weight training!** You don't just stop at 12 repetitions because that's your number to stop. "Going to fatigue" means that you *can't do any more*. More specifically, you can't continue in *good form*. For instance, if you find that you start throwing your body around, arching your back, or using momentum to complete an exercise, it's time to stop. You could do more harm than good at that point. For this reason, it is often helpful to have a full-body mirror available while you do your weight-training program. A mirror is a great tool to use for monitoring your form.

Progressing

Figuring out what weight will get you to fatigue within 8–15 repetitions is a work in progress. Sometimes, you over-estimate or underestimate the correct weight that will cause fatigue for, let's say, 12 repetitions. If you complete 11 repetitions one day, that's fine. If it's 14 another day, that's fine, too. When you are consistently able to do more than 15, it's time to try a heavier weight. If you can get past 8 reps in good form with the higher weight, it's a keeper. Then, as you stay with that weight, you'll work your way back up to 12 reps again. Over more weeks and months, you may start creeping up towards 15 reps again, signaling that it's time to again try a heavier weight. If you always concentrate on "going to fatigue", you will always get maximum benefit out of the exercise.

> **Time out please—**
> **my brain is on overload**
>
> "This seems like a lot of details. I'm not sure I care about all this."
>
> "Oh, if I'm going to do one of the less intense exercise levels, I won't need to worry about all this info? Thanks! I'll skim past it."

Sets

Once you complete your desired number of repetitions, you have completed one set. You may or may not do another set after resting that muscle group for a few minutes. For example, if you perform 12 repetitions of the bicep curl exercise, rest for a few minutes and then do 12 more, you have just completed two sets of bicep curls.

How Many Sets?

Most general fitness enthusiasts will do 1–3 sets per muscle group. One set is the perfect place to start and is also where many people stay—it's quick and still beneficial. Two sets will give even more benefits, and three even more than that. There's no reason to feel locked into a particular program. Let it change and evolve as you have more and less time. If you know more than one exercise for each muscle group, you may want to mix it up even more, as long as you generally do the same number of sets for each muscle group. For instance, push-ups and dumbbell flies both work the chest muscles. If you typically do two sets per muscle group, you may decide to do two sets of push-ups, two sets of flies, or one set of each. The choice is yours and variety is a good thing. Your body responds well to surprises!

How Often?

The general rule of thumb is to do your strength-training program three times per week—always with a day off in between. A more modest program may be twice a week and that is still beneficial. Remember that during your workout, you are microscopically shredding your muscle cells; they need about 48 hours to repair themselves and grow stronger. That's why you generally skip a day between weight-training workouts.

How Long Will It Take?

The good news is that your entire routine could take as little as five to ten minutes or as long as an hour, depending on the number of sets per muscle group, which in turn is dependent upon your goals, time available, and enthusiasm. Remember, it's flexible and whether it's minimal or extensive, it's worthwhile!

A Summary of Resistance Training Principles:
- 2–3 times per week (always skip a day between)
- 1–3 sets per body part
- 8–15 repetitions per set
- Select the weight that will cause fatigue within 8–15 repetitions
- If you're not at fatigue by the end of your predetermined range of repetitions, keep going until you do reach fatigue and consider increasing the weight next time.

You should feel pretty confident that you now know enough about strength training to get to the next step—selecting your routine in the next section.

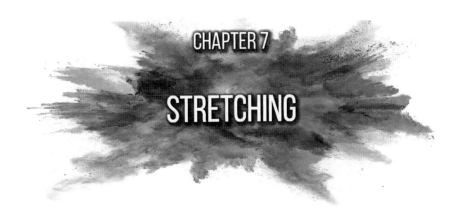

CHAPTER 7

STRETCHING

FLEXIBILITY IS THE ability of your muscles to go through a full range of motion. There is a genetic component that we all come to realize starting in childhood. Even as adults, if you were asked to touch your toes, most people know in advance whether they'd be successful. Maximizing your flexibility is especially important for those who aren't naturally flexible and yet, this same population typically avoids it the most.

You won't be able to *see* the benefits of stretching, but you will *feel* them. Increased flexibility helps keep your muscles limber and receptive to reaching, bending, and comfortably participating in a variety of activities. It can also be helpful for preventing injuries, such as muscle strains. Stretching can also provide relief for stress-induced muscle tension and help rehabilitate any number of overuse injuries.

You can improve your flexibility by doing stretching exercises. Stretches are best performed slowly and gently to the point of mild tension and then held in that position. There are specific positions that stretch each major muscle group. An example would be lying on the floor on your back and holding your knees into your chest. This position stretches your lower back muscles

Here are some tips to keep in mind about stretching:

- Remember that flexibility is specific to each muscle group. For a complete program, you'll need to do a series of stretches, each targeting a different muscle group.

- Flexibility is different in each person and is determined largely by genetics. Don't compare yourself to others with regard to how far you can stretch. Concentrate on stretching correctly and to the point that your body can comfortably reach.

- You should stretch slowly and gently to the point of mild tension (not pain) and then hold that position.

- Hold a stretch for 15–30 seconds for a mild stretch and up to a minute or more if you are trying to improve a particular problem with a muscle.

- Don't bounce when you stretch. Think about what happens when you quickly stretch a rubber band. A quick, forceful stretch on the rubber does not result in a lengthened rubber band. Instead, it snaps back. This is a great analogy for your muscles and is the opposite of what you want. Gently ease into a slow, gradual stretch.

- Stretching and warming up are not the same thing. Warming up involves doing some form of light activity (like walking or bicycling) for 3–5 minutes, which increases your circulation and body temperature to prepare your body for your workout. Stretching may also be done before your aerobic or strength training workout, but only after your warm-up. Once your circulation has increased and your muscles are warmer, they are softer and more pliable, making them more receptive to stretching. This is why you may have been told to avoid stretching when your muscles are cold.

- Stretching is most effective for increasing flexibility when done after your workout when your muscles are at their warmest.

- Try to stretch a minimum of three times per week in order to gain the most benefits. If you enjoy it, stretching exercises can safely be done every day. In fact, if you are recovering from a chronic muscle injury, your doctor or physical therapist might prescribe stretching exercises to be done 3–5 times per day.

- Not every stretch will feel good for everybody. Try out a new stretch gently for the first time to see if it's comfortable for you. Also, be sure to seek professional guidance from a fitness trainer if you are unsure about correct positioning or appropriateness of a particular stretch for you.

STRETCHING IS SUPER!

A regular stretching program will take you far in comfort and ease of movement during everyday life and as you age. Even though everyone's genetic potential for flexibility is different, most of us are not reaching our potential. Years of disuse cause our muscles to shorten unnecessarily, creating an overall stiffness and a breeding ground for all sorts of aches and pains. Make sure you don't fall into the trap of using "I've never been flexible," as an excuse not to stretch. A simple stretching routine several times per week can make a big difference for anyone. You can improve your flexibility and it is well worth it!

TIME FOR A STRETCH BREAK!

Anytime you need to improve your mood, reduce fatigue, and ease stiff, achy muscles, try this *"Quick Stretch Break Sequence"* which stretches the upper back, shoulders, chest, neck, biceps, and triceps. Hold each position for 10-30 seconds before moving to the next step. If any position causes pain, discontinue that portion of the routine.

1. Clasp your hands out in front of you with straight arms and press out, rounding your upper back.

2. Slowly raise your arms, hands still clasped together, above your head and press up.

3. Release your clasped hands; grab one wrist and tug upward. Change and grab the other wrist and tug upward.

4. Bring your arms down and place your hands on the back of your head. Pull your elbows back, squeezing your shoulder blades together.

5. Let your arms fall open, straightening your elbows with your palms facing up.

6. Press your arms down and out through the heel of your hands. Drop your head slowly to one side, then circle halfway around to the other side.

7. Lift one arm overhead, elbow bent, with your hand hanging down your back. With the fingertips of your opposite hand, pull back at the elbow. Switch.

Give stretching a try! You'll be glad you did!

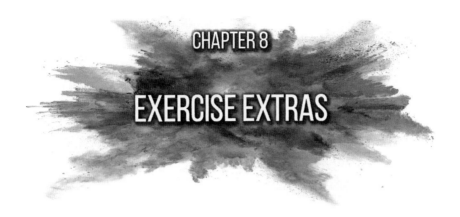

CHAPTER 8

EXERCISE EXTRAS

WHAT ABOUT YOGA, **Pilates, and Tai Chi?**
There are other valuable and popular kinds of exercise that do not neatly fall into one of the three categories of aerobic exercise, strength training, and stretching. Rather, they give some benefit in several categories and offer great appeal to many people.

Yoga, tai chi, and Pilates have many similarities. All three deliver significant flexibility and strength benefits, but do not typically have a direct influence on cardiovascular fitness. Yoga and tai chi are both particularly good for helping improve balance, flexibility, posture, brain health and can be a calming source of relaxation and stress management. They are worth looking into if you find these practices enjoyable.

NEVER TOO EARLY
Extras

If any of these extras interest you, go for it!

NEVER TOO LATE
Extras

Balance is super important! Make sure you address this to decrease your risk of falls. Tai Chi is fantastic for this. If regular Yoga is too strenuous, look for a seated yoga class.

Balance

Poor balance as we age can come from a combination of sources: inner ear conditions, vision problems, numbness in the feet and legs, heart or circulation problems, medication interactions, and certain diseases like Alzheimer's, Parkinson's disease, and Multiple Sclerosis. The most significant cause of balance issues however is the gradual loss of muscle over the years due to reduced activity. **This means that the number one strategy to improve balance is to increase leg strength.**

That being said, *balance* has become almost a separate fitness component to consider as we age. You will often see balance classes and articles specifically outlining balance exercises in an effort to prevent falls in older adults, which can be deadly. These can be very helpful and yet I would not advise choosing balance exercises over strength training, but rather in addition to it.

Putting It All Together

We've covered the basics in the areas of aerobic exercise, strength training, and stretching. Now it's time to take a quick look at a few other considerations to keep in mind when embarking on a new fitness lifestyle.

Health History

How's your health? It's important to check with your doctor before starting a vigorous exercise routine if you are over the age of 45, have heart or lung problems, diabetes, bone or joint problems, or several of the risk factors for cardiovascular disease. Even given the above, in most cases, your doctor is still going to be in favor of you beginning an exercise program. He or she may, however, have specific recommendations for you and/or may want to supervise your efforts more closely. Please don't let this be a deterrent to getting started. Your body needs to exercise! You'll be glad you followed up.

Warm-Up

It is important to ease your body into exercise. Whether you are about to do aerobic exercise, strength training, or stretching, spending 3–5 minutes walking or doing some other form of light continuous movement is important to warm up. (Remember that warming up literally means increasing your body temperature and that warming up and stretching are not the same thing.) In this way, you'll prepare your body for exercise by increasing circulation to your muscles that will soon need it.

Cool-Down

Cool-down applies specifically to aerobic exercise. It is recommended that you take 3-5 minutes at the end of your aerobic workout to walk slowly or simply do a lower intensity version of whatever activity you were doing. This will allow your heart rate to gradually slow back to a normal rate. Abruptly stopping your aerobic workout while you are at a high intensity can lead to dizziness or tingling legs as the blood tries to climb back up to the brain against gravity without the help of your muscles continuing to contract. For people who are at a high risk for heart disease, the absence of a cool-down period can result in irregular heartbeats or other cardiac rhythm irregularities. Don't forget to cool down!

A Few Extra Tips

- Buy good shoes. You need adequate arch support, cushioning, and stability in your athletic shoes. When you are serious about fitness, treat your feet right to avoid injuries.

- Receive proper instruction. This book contains detailed recommendations for many exercise options, however, if you have any questions about what is right and appropriate for you, please consult with a fitness trainer.

He or she can make sure that you are performing all of your exercises properly so that you don't injure yourself and are gaining maximum benefits.

- Listen to your body. Exercise should not hurt. All exercises are not right for all people. If something hurts or doesn't feel comfortable, that's your cue to stop. Pushing yourself is expected, but when your body says, "Enough," you should listen.

- Have fun! Remember, as you try to decide what is going to be the right exercise plan for you, if it isn't fun, chances are you won't be able to stick with it. We're trying to build a lifestyle that includes fitness. What can you see as part of your life?

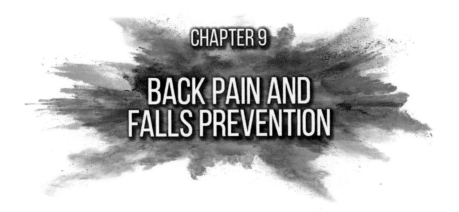

CHAPTER 9

BACK PAIN AND FALLS PREVENTION

B ACK PAIN AND falls prevention are two important and very common concerns that only increase as we age; the good news is that they are especially improved by exercise. Let's take a special look at these two areas. The specific exercises that help them are rolled into the exercise levels in the next section.

BACK PAIN

Your body will not feel very strong or energetic if you have back pain. Unfortunately, approximately 80% of adults suffer from back pain at some point in their lives, yet only 10% of those who suffer find out the primary cause. Some statistics say that over $50 billion is spent on back pain treatment each year and over $100 billion in indirect costs!

Back pain has become so common that many people think it's "normal" and they default to thinking they have a "bad back". When back pain is viewed as a medical problem that needs medical treatment, we miss the opportunity to realize that many back problems are due to biomechanical and muscular imbalance issues that arise from our sedentary lives. Weak abdominal muscles, excess weight, and tight lower back muscles often cause undue strain on the lower back.

Did you know that many cases of lower back pain are caused by weak abdominal muscles? That's right—weak, sagging abdominal muscles can tug the pelvis down, tilting it forward. This forward pelvic tilt can cause the lower back muscles to tighten when you want them to be stretched and relaxed.

Take a look at the muscles surrounding the pelvis in the illustration below. The abdominal muscles and the gluteus maximus muscles work together to tilt the pelvis forward or back. When the abdominal and gluteal muscles are strong (as in the darkly shaded illustration on the left), they tilt the pelvis backwards. The back is less arched and there is no back pain. When the abdominal and gluteal muscles are weak (as in the lightly shaded illustration on the right), they are not strong enough to tilt the pelvis back, so the pelvis tilts forward. Excess weight causes the pelvis to tilt forward even more. This forward pelvic tilt accentuates the arch in the lower back with tighter lower back muscles and back pain.

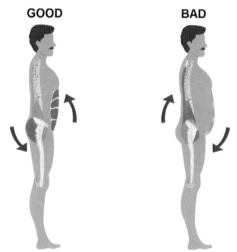

GOOD   BAD

If weak abdominal muscles and overly tight lower back muscles are a primary contributor to lower back pain, then the natural two-part remedy is to:
- Strengthen the abdominal muscles, and
- Stretch the lower back muscles.

Below are two lower back pain exercise routines: "NEVER TOO EARLY" is for those who are on the younger side and/or more mobile and able to get down and up off the floor. "NEVER TOO LATE" is for those who are a bit older in age and/or have limited mobility, health concerns, or are not comfortable getting down and up off the floor.

NEVER TOO EARLY

Plank

Start on the floor lying on your stomach. Come up on your toes and forearms, keeping your body completely straight (don't let your hips sag down or pike up). If you find that this position is too intense, you can do the modified version on your toes and hands. Consciously hold your abdominal muscles in tightly. The goal is to stay in this position for as long as possible. At first, this could be just a few seconds, but you will want to build up to 60 seconds or more.

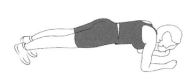 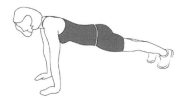

Lower Back Stretch

Lie on your back on the floor and pull both knees to your chest, clasping your hands under your knees if possible. Hold this position for at least 30 seconds, or as long as several minutes if you have chronic lower back pain. If you can only hold it for 30 seconds, repeat it several times.

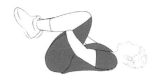

NEVER TOO LATE

Seated Abdominal Crunch

This abdominal strengthening exercise is perfect for those who are not comfortable getting down and up from the floor. In the starting position, you are sitting close to the edge of the chair and straight up. Slowly lean back until you *almost* touch your shoulder blades to the back of the chair. You should feel your abdominal muscles tighten. Then slowly come back up to starting position again.

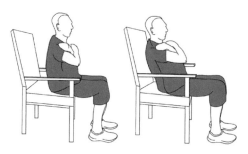

Seated Lower Back Stretch

Version 1—With Rounded Spine: While seated, simply place your feet shoulder-width apart, round your back over, and let your head and hands lower down. Stay in this position for 15-30 seconds. Your lower back muscles will relax and lengthen.

Version 2—With Straight Spine: If you have osteoporosis, lean forward with a straight spine while keeping your hands on your thighs and do not lower your head below your knees.

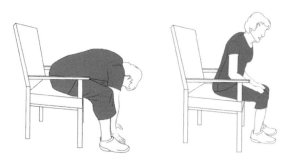

Whether you do the "Never Too Early" or "Never Too Late" version of these exercises, they should take just a few minutes per day. Try them three or more times per week and you'll see a difference in how your back feels!

Of course, there are other things that will also help reduce and prevent lower back pain.

1. *Less sitting*
    When most people sit, they tend to slouch and allow the abdominal muscles to overly relax. In addition, people who sit for long periods of time are not moving around enough during the day to combat the effects of sitting.

2. *More moving and more walking*
    Whenever you move or walk, your body needs to at least slightly contract your abdominal muscles to maintain your upright posture. You also need to use your gluteal muscles a bit and this increased overall activity helps keep all the muscles around the pelvis stronger than they would otherwise be.

3. *Better posture*
    Those who are conscious of standing tall, holding their shoulders back and abdominal muscles in have a natural advantage in warding off back pain. Great posture involves all-day muscle engagement which is excellent for back pain prevention.

4. *Lose weight*
    Excess weight, especially in the abdominal region pulls the pelvis forward and out of alignment. This additional strain forces the lower back muscles to become overly tight and elicits pain. Imagine holding a 25-pound dumbbell at your waist and walking around all day to get an idea of the extra strain that is on your muscles all day long when you carry even 25 extra pounds on your frame.

5. *Aerobic exercise*
Whether you are walking, enjoying water exercise, or an elliptical machine, any form of aerobic exercise engages your abdominal muscles and other major muscle groups for stabilization and helps keep them strong to avoid back pain.

6. *General weight training*
You don't need to be doing abdominal muscle exercises specifically in order for your abdominal muscles to contract. As with aerobic exercise, general weight training engages your abdominal muscles and other major muscle groups to stabilize the body and give them an added workout that helps prevent back pain.

FALLS PREVENTION

Falls prevention is an important issue as we age—and with good reason. For older adults, a fall could lead to a broken bone or other injury that would be an inconvenience at best and a serious health set-back at worst. In fact, according to the Center for Disease Control (CDC), falls are the *leading cause* of fatal injury and the most common cause of nonfatal trauma-related hospital admissions among older adults. Here are some staggering statistics about falls from the CDC:

- One in four Americans aged 65+ falls each year
- Every eleven seconds, an older adult is treated in the emergency room for a fall; every nineteen minutes, an older adult dies from a fall.
- Falls result in more than 2.8 million injuries treated in emergency departments annually, including over 800,000 hospitalizations and more than 27,000 deaths.
- In 2015, the total cost of fall injuries was $50 billion. Medicare and Medicaid shouldered 75% of these costs.

- The financial toll for older adult falls is expected to increase over the coming years as the population ages.

Wow! Falls are clearly a risk to be taken seriously. The good news is that there is much we can do to reduce our risk.

NEVER TOO EARLY

In your younger years, if you experience a fall, you are less likely to experience a fracture or serious injury, but now is the time to maintain your strength and flexibility. If you are not already in the habit of a strength-training routine, start now. Work to keep your leg muscles (quadriceps) strong to avoid the dreaded loss of 50% of your leg strength by the time you are eighty years old that we talked about in the beginning of this book. This is your *best* strategy to protect your older self. Start now!

NEVER TOO LATE

There are some basic strategies that go a long way in reducing your risk of experiencing a fall. None are time consuming. All are worthwhile when you consider the possible devastating effects of a fall. The first one is EXERCISE! (Surprised?) This is because:

1. One of the most important factors in falls prevention is **BALANCE.**
2. One of the most important factors in good balance is **LEG STRENGTH.**
3. One of the best ways to improve leg strength is with the **"SIT-TO-STAND" exercise**.

Sit-to-Stand

The Sit-to-Stand exercise is simple to do and requires only a sturdy chair. The movement is quite straightforward: stand up and sit back down without using your arms to assist.

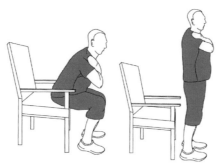

A few tips for doing this exercise:

- Make sure the chair is sturdy (no wheels and not a flimsy chair). Push the chair up against a wall for maximum stability.

- How many? To test yourself, see how many Sit-to-Stand repetitions you can do in 30 seconds.

  o If you are unable to do even one repetition, it would be unsafe to proceed with this specific exercise, but it means that strengthening your leg muscles is that much more necessary. Start with a different leg-strengthening exercise: the seated leg extension. Stay seated, lift one leg up, and then bend and extend at the knee. Start with just a few on each side and work up to 20 or more repetitions on each leg. You can also add ankle weights if it's too easy.

  o If you can do more than one but less than 10 repetitions, start with whatever amount you can do and then gradually build up to 10-20 or more. If you need a little help from your upper body to push off the chair or to hold onto a railing, that's okay in the beginning, but the goal is to gradually be able to perform the exercise unassisted. You will get there if you do the exercise consistently!

  o If you can do 10 or more repetitions, continue to do as many as you can daily to maintain and build your strength.

o   If you can do 30 or more, consider contacting a fitness professional for a more challenging exercise routine.

The Leg Extension

The Leg Extension is for you if you are unable to perform the Sit-to-Stand for even one repetition. Sit upright in a chair and lift one leg so that the knee is a bit higher than the other leg. Kick out your foot until your knee is straight and then bend it to return to the starting position. If you don't keep your moving knee a bit higher than the stationary knee, your foot will bump into the floor and stop your range of motion before you fully return to the starting position. Perform 8–12 repetitions for each leg.

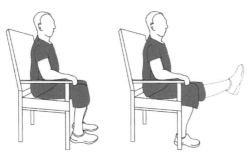

Additional Steps to Take to Reduce Your Risk of Falling

- Make sure your vision is good.
- Be aware of medications that may cause dizziness.
- Take your time—don't rush when walking.
- Wear safety-conscious, sturdy shoes with non-slip soles.
- Consider the conditions—and stay inside in rainy, icy conditions.
- Watch for slip hazards such as rugs without non-slip backings, and clutter.
- Use a nightlight at night.
- Walk with confidence. The fear of falling increases your risk of falling!

Better safe than sorry!

STEP THREE:

THE **BOOM** FITNESS FRAMEWORK AND EXERCISE LEVELS

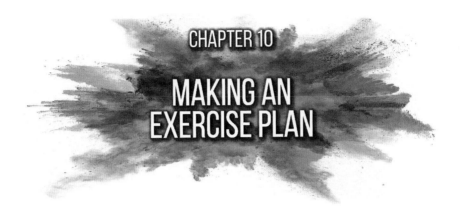

CHAPTER 10

MAKING AN EXERCISE PLAN

YOU HAVE MANY OPTIONS

THE NEXT QUESTION becomes, "How can I decide what is the right kind, amount, and intensity of exercise for me?" In the following chapters, I'll give you a variety of scenarios from which to choose. You may end up creating your own program after checking out the options in this book and that is fine. Remember, the goal is to find the program that is going to get you active over the long term. Everybody can find some form and amount of exercise that will fit their schedule. It doesn't have to be a lot, but it does have to be consistent to impact your body, brain, and energy levels. Slow and steady wins the race. Let's look at some of your options.

THE BOOM FITNESS FRAMEWORK WITH FOUR EXERCISE LEVELS

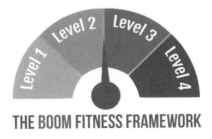

THE BOOM FITNESS FRAMEWORK

Placing a framework around your efforts is the path to consistency, so let's allow for options that take a minimalist approach all the way up to a comprehensive plan. There are four levels to the BOOM Fitness Framework and for each level, there is an option for NEVER TOO EARLY and NEVER TOO LATE. Remember that whether the NEVER TOO EARLY or NEVER TOO LATE track is right for you is not determined solely by your age. You will also consider your exercise history, overall health and energy level, and any special concerns that might warrant a more conservative approach versus a more rigorous approach.

The main difference between the levels is how much time you are willing to devote to your exercise routine. We'll devote an entire chapter to each level, addressing both the NEVER TOO EARLY and NEVER TOO LATE options within that level. Level 1 is entitled "Just MOVE", designed for those not interested in structured exercise, but who admit they need to be more active. Level 2 is a home-based 20-minute minimalist approach that doesn't require any equipment, but is a bit more structured than "Just MOVE".

Level 3 is also home-based, but it's a little longer, including a 40-minute moderate level commitment that offers even more benefits than the earlier levels and requires a few inexpensive pieces of exercise equipment.

Finally, there is Level 4 that is appropriate for those who wish to go "all out". If you fall into this category, you will likely already have resources to assist you in the development of your routine. Specific routines for Level 4 are beyond the scope of this book, however we will address it briefly. It is very common for individuals to work their way up to a Level 4 commitment over time.

Hands-on assistance from a certified fitness professional is wise to make sure you learn the correct exercises and form that is right for you. Your job is to select the level and track that feels like a good fit for you right now based on your health, schedule, frame of mind, and current goals.

The BOOM Fitness Framework		
Level	NEVER TOO EARLY Track	NEVER TOO LATE Track
1	Just MOVE	Just MOVE
2	20-Minute No Equipment Home Exercise Plan	20-Minute No Equipment Home Exercise Plan
3	40-Minute Minimal Equipment Home Exercise Plan	40-Minute Minimal Equipment Home Exercise Plan
4	60-Minute+ Full-Fledged Program Specific routines for this level are beyond the scope of this book. You can get the best advice from a certified fitness trainer or staff at your local fitness center.	60-minute+ Full-Fledged Program Specific routines for this level are beyond the scope of this book. You can get the best advice from a certified fitness trainer or staff at your local fitness center. Look for a trainer who specializes in older adults.

The Exercise Levels are Fluid

One of the most important features of the levels and the tracks is that they are fluid. They are not meant to put you in a box and keep you there. Choosing the 20-Minute Plan, for instance, simply means that your time, commitment and interest level matches this plan right now. You don't necessarily ever have to graduate to the next level.

You will probably find that you'll slide back and forth through the different levels as your time, fitness level, and enthusiasm rises and falls. You may slide back and forth due to travel, the seasons, illness, or family commitments. A shift back and forth may be over a period of weeks or months, or all in the same week. There is no rule that says you can't have one workout each week from each of the categories.

Remember that the goal is consistency. In permitting yourself to slide back and forth between these levels, you will eliminate stopping altogether as an option—and the guilt that comes with it.

Look at the levels illustrated as "positions on the dial". The levels can blur seamlessly one into the next, giving you the opportunity to choose something in between the levels if you wish. Only you can decide when or if it's time for you to "turn up the dial"!

Tips for Choosing the Exercise Level that is Right for You

- Build a strong base with daily movement.
- Each level on the dial represents a progressively more comprehensive approach.
- Choose your level based on your time constraints, commitment level, and interest.
- The levels are flexible and fluid. Feel free to take it up or down a notch on the dial based on changes in your schedule and interest.
- More is better than less, but some is better than none.
- You be the judge on what level best fits you.
- Choosing none is not an option!

AN OVERVIEW OF THE LEVELS

Remember that there is a NEVER TOO EARLY and a NEVER TOO LATE track for each level.

Level 1: Just MOVE!

Accumulate 30 minutes of intentional movement on most days. It does not need to be all at one time. It can be broken up throughout the day.

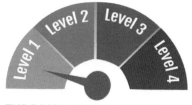

THE BOOM FITNESS FRAMEWORK

The Benefits

There are significant long-term health benefits in your future if you adopt a lifestyle of moving more, especially doing so intentionally for 30 minutes per day, including:

- Improved general health.
- Increased energy.
- Reduced risk of a host of chronic diseases—heart disease, diabetes, and some cancers.
- Increased calorie burning from more activity.
- A positive experience of not biting off more than you can chew and burning out.
- Consistency with an intentional effort toward fitness.
- A fitness-conscious mindset that may lead to a lifetime of exercise.

Worthwhile benefits, aren't they?!

Level 2: The 20-Minute No Equipment Home Exercise Plan (3 times per week)

- 15 minutes of walking (you can start and end right at your own front door) or another cardio-vascular exercise
- One Abdominal Strengthening Exercise
- One Upper Body Strengthening Exercise
- One Lower Body Strengthening Exercise
- Lower Back Stretch

THE BOOM FITNESS FRAMEWORK

The Benefits
Look at all you will be doing for yourself by adopting this level of exercise:

- All the benefits listed in Level 1 (but to a larger degree), plus—
- Increased strength in your core, legs, chest, and arms.
- Improved brain health and mental clarity.
- Improved strength and capacity of your heart and lungs.

- Improved blood pressure.
- An outlet for stress.
- Improved sleep patterns.
- Increased metabolic rate.
- Stronger and more taut abdominal muscles leading to improved appearance.
- Alleviation or prevention of lower back pain.
- A sense of accomplishment and possibly a desire for more exercise down the road.

Wow! That's some list for a quick 20 minutes, isn't it?!

Level 3: The 40-Minute Minimal Equipment Home Exercise Plan (3–4 times per week)

- 20 minutes of your choice of aerobic exercise 3-4 times per week (walking, jogging, elliptical machine, stationary bicycle, NuStep machine, or swimming)

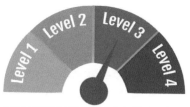

THE BOOM FITNESS FRAMEWORK

- A short (<20 minute) weight-training routine, 3 times per week (one set of one exercise per muscle group)
- Several stretching exercises for key muscle groups

The Benefits
Onward and upward with the cumulative benefits as you work through the levels! The benefits of the 40-Minute Plan are truly fantastic! Take a look:

- All the benefits listed in Level 2, but to a larger degree! More exercise and increased rigor of the routine will increase the level of benefit you receive from each of the following points listed. Good for you!

Plus:

- Noticeably increased muscular strength and endurance for all your major muscle groups.
- An even greater increase in metabolic rate.
- Even greater improvement in aerobic capacity and cardiovascular endurance.
- Help with weight loss due to more substantial increases in metabolism and calorie burning.
- Knowledge and practice in knowing what makes up a comprehensive strength training routine, making for an easy transition to the Full-Fledged Plan should you decide to do that at some point.

Level 4: The 60-Minute+ Full-Fledged Exercise Plan (3–6 times per week)

- 20–60 minutes of varied aerobic exercise, 3–5 times per week (walking, jogging, elliptical machine, or stationary bicycle)
- A 20–40-minute weight-training routine, 3 times per week (2–3 sets per muscle group)
- Stretching exercises for each major muscle group

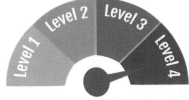

THE BOOM FITNESS FRAMEWORK

The Benefits
All the benefits listed in Level 3, but to an even larger degree! Once again, a more rigorous and comprehensive routine will increase the level of benefit you receive. Fantastic!

SAFETY TIPS

1. Always stop if you feel dizzy, extremely short of breath, nauseous, shaky, or if you experience pain or tightness in your throat or chest.

2. If a certain exercise causes pain, stop doing it and don't do that exercise again. It is important to learn the difference between tired muscles and pain. There is also a difference between normal muscle soreness after exercise and harmful pain. Pain in a joint means "stop"; mild discomfort in the muscles means that you are working your muscles correctly.

3. Mild muscle soreness one to two days after working out (especially after new exercise) is normal and to be expected. Take it easy for a few days to allow the soreness to subside. Then, resume your exercise routine. Likely, the soreness will decrease after the next few workouts, once your body is used to it.

4. Use good posture during exercise and avoid locking your joints.

5. Avoid fast, jerky movements. Try for gentle, smooth movements.

6. Never hold your breath during exercise. Breathe naturally.

7. Listen to your body. Stop when you feel as though you've had enough.

WHAT'S NEXT?

Once you are living the flexible exercise level lifestyle, enjoy it and see where it takes you. You may be content to keep your routine consistent, just as many of us are content to eat the same thing for breakfast or lunch every day. Others crave variety and feel the need to change things more often. For instance, after having a certain pattern for three or six months, you may find yourself becoming bored. If that's you, start looking around for ways to change things up.

Your ears might perk up about an upcoming long-distance walk for charity. Training for that walk becomes your focal point. You'll meet new people and have a great sense of accomplishment. You may decide to hire a personal trainer for a few sessions to pick up some new exercise ideas. You may also check out the local gym and start mixing some exercise classes into your usually solo exercise habits. You might decide it's finally time to invest in a little more substantial home exercise equipment. There are many ideas for the taking! Go for it!

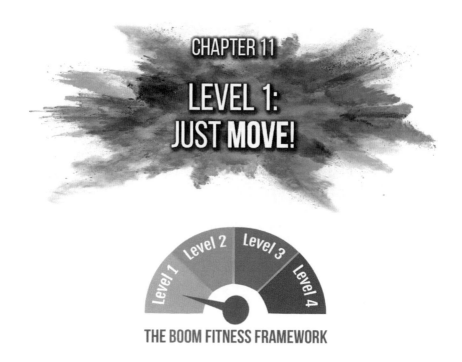

CHAPTER 11
LEVEL 1:
JUST MOVE!

THE BOOM FITNESS FRAMEWORK

DAILY ACTIVITY ADDS UP

A MEANINGFUL MOVEMENT goal is to simply add more activity to your existing daily life because it truly does add up.

This might be a good strategy for you if:

- You feel "allergic to exercise"—don't like it, never did, and don't see it changing anytime soon.
- You've never liked to sweat.
- You can't see where or how you'd set aside a specific recurring time to exercise.
- You don't really want to set aside a specific recurring time to exercise.
- You don't see yourself changing into exercise clothes to work out.

To quantify it somewhat, try to accumulate 30 minutes of activity on most days, above what you normally do. It doesn't have to be all at once. It can be interspersed throughout the day. Sounds too simple? Sounds too insignificant? Think again.

While you consider how daily activity adds up, don't forget that it is beneficial for everyone. Even those who have rigorous exercise routines benefit from increasing daily activity during the rest of the day.

We all know that it is good to be more active rather than less active. Our bodies thrive on movement, yet many of us spend just a few too many hours in front of the TV or computer. When we do think about activity, most of us think automatically about structured exercise—the kind that is on purpose, while wearing exercise clothing . . . the kind that we don't have time for.

Think again—this time about the little things that make up an active lifestyle and make a difference! You know those tips such as "park farther away" or "take the stairs instead of the elevator"? If you're like most people, you may be secretly thinking, "That stuff can't possibly make a difference." Actually, that stuff does make a difference. And here's why:

> Our bodies are calorie-burning machines 24 hours a day. Even if you exercised one full hour per day (which is a lot), there are still 23 hours of metabolic activity to be accounted for. If you don't give a second thought to your activity level throughout the day, you are missing a great opportunity to have a huge impact on your health, your metabolism, and your body weight. What is your body doing during the other twenty-three hours per day?

ALL IN A DAY'S WORK . . . OR LACK THEREOF

The average person burns approximately one calorie per minute, sitting at rest. The same person, while standing, will burn 1.5

calories per minute. You may be thinking "an extra half calorie—big deal." While it may not be a big deal for one minute, or even one hour, burning 50% more calories while standing instead of sitting is a pretty big deal when you spend a good part of your day sitting instead of standing!

Walking at a leisurely pace burns approximately two calories per minute—double that of sitting. Aerobic exercise, such as brisk walking or jogging can burn up to 8–12 calories per minute. That's why aerobic exercise is a great way to burn a sizeable extra chunk of calories per day and can help with weight loss. But, since aerobic exercise isn't realistically going to account for a very big part of your day, it's a good idea to give some thought to the daily activities that make up the other 23 hours of the day. They truly add up!

AND THE DAYS TURN INTO WEEKS

Let's take it one step further to give some thought to your metabolic activity in an entire week. There are 168 hours in a week. Using our example of a person who exercises for a full hour each day, there are still 161 hours (or 96%) of the week to consider. Can you think of any other area in your life in which you'd like to make an improvement and chose to ignore 96% of the time available to you?

Keep in mind how our labor-saving and time-saving culture robs us of opportunities to use our bodies. Think about drive-thru fast food, circling for the closest spot (even if it takes longer), waiting and waiting for the elevator instead of taking the stairs, ride-on lawn mowers, and emailing or texting someone sitting just down the hall. Physical labor used to be part of the average American's day, but it is no more. You can turn that around! Choose the more active option rather than the less active option when possible. Seek out ways to use your body rather than ways to save energy.

TAKING ACTION

Armed with the reasons why, let's take another look at the tried-and-true suggestions below. I like to think of these techniques as "sneaking exercise" into your day. Think of all the little things that separately seem insignificant, but together, can make a big difference:

- Stand rather than sit when you can.
- Take the stairs instead of the elevator.
- Park at the far end of the parking lot.
- Get off the metro one stop early and walk the rest of the way.
- Stand up while talking on the phone.
- Walk down the hall at the office to deliver a message in person.
- Go up and down the stairs in your home frequently rather than making a pile at the bottom of the stairs to bring up later.

MAKE IT A CONSCIOUS, INTENTIONAL DECISION

You may already be moving around a good bit during the day, but you're not sure exactly how much, and you know you can do better. Why not try to be a little more intentional to take it to the next level? Here are some ideas for holding yourself accountable for your goal of accumulating thirty minutes or more of activity on most days. It will seem more concrete if you make specific decisions and try to reset your patterns. "Vague" rarely works. Be specific and you'll see changes happen.

Which of the following thought patterns do you think will most likely lead to success?

> *"I'll try to take the stairs more often instead of the elevator."*

> *"I will take the stairs Monday through Friday when I go to the cafeteria at lunchtime."*

How about these two choices?

"I'll try to walk more often throughout the day."

"Every time I go shopping, I'll park at the far end of the lot to make for a longer walk to the front door."

MAKE A PLAN

Break up the 30 minutes into three 10-minute exercise bites throughout the day. Find some small way to increase the movement involved in something that's already part of your morning, afternoon, and/or evening routine. Maybe you'll plan a quick 10-minute mini-walk in the morning, at lunch, and in the evening. How about getting a dog? People who have dogs usually get more exercise than those who don't, since the dog needs to be walked (and so do you)!

COUNT YOUR STEPS

Pedometers, Fitbits, Apple Watches, and apps on your phone are all great tools to get a better idea of how much you are moving each day. You can see that specific goals make this technique come to life. Many of them also track distance covered in miles or kilometers, total calories burned, and many other interesting facts. A study in JAMA (the *Journal of the American Medical Association*) found that simply giving someone a pedometer caused their activity level to increase by 25%!

You may have heard that a good goal for overall health if you are going to track your steps, is taking 10,000 steps per day. If that seems like a whole lot more than you are currently doing, take an incremental approach. Test your average number of steps during what would be a normal day for you and then set a goal of perhaps 500-1,000 additional steps. Depending on your unique circumstances, you may be able to keep bumping up your goal to eventually get to 10,000 steps.

If not, you will still be doing a great thing for your health by increasing your steps to the extent that works for you. Remember, we're trying to create long-term habits. There's no need to rush into anything. You will find over time that you'll probably need to do some intentional activity to get up to 10,000 steps per day. Get creative and keep using the pedometer for a while. Raising your consciousness is what's going to make a difference. Once you get into the habit, there may come a time when you find you don't need to wear it to approximate your activity anymore, unless you enjoy it.

LEVEL 1

NEVER TOO EARLY

Let your motivation be your guide! Level 1 is a great way to build some movement into your life and the 10,000-step goal should certainly be within reach. The upper limits of what is described in this chapter are meant for you—test yourself and see how it can grow!

NEVER TOO LATE

As you read through the chapter, you'll see references to starting slow and basing your goals on incremental increases to what you are currently doing. Ten thousand steps per day will likely be unreasonable if you have mobility issues, and therefore you'd want to see what you are currently doing and set a goal for a bit more than that.

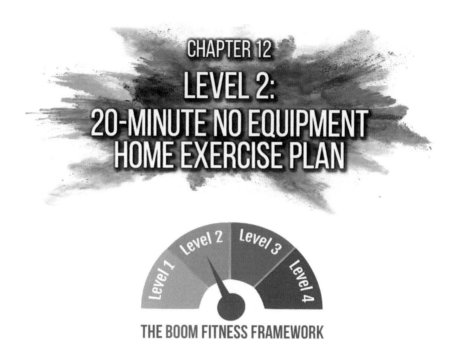

CHAPTER 12
LEVEL 2:
20-MINUTE NO EQUIPMENT
HOME EXERCISE PLAN

THE BOOM FITNESS FRAMEWORK

YOU'VE DECIDED THAT you'd like to commit to exercising on purpose several times per week, but still think a minimalist approach is the way to go, at least for now. Bravo! You'll need to plan for 20 minutes of intentional exercise all at once, 3 times per week. Your 20-minute workout will include:

- 15 minutes of cardiovascular exercise (walking or using a cardiovascular machine)
- One abdominal strengthening exercise
- One upper body strengthening exercise
- One lower body strengthening exercise
- One stretching exercise—lower back stretch

Why did I select these exercises? In just 20 minutes of intentional exercise, this routine will allow you to address each of the three categories of exercise: aerobic exercise, strength training, and stretching. For the strength training portion, you will target one upper body muscle group, one lower body muscle group, plus your abdominals, which is a respectable bare minimum approach for an intentional exercise session. It is especially valuable to focus on your abdominal muscles.

Popular fitness lingo refers to this muscle group as part of your "core", which provides your body's overall stability. Strong abdominal muscles help with posture, prevent lower back pain, and improve your appearance. A lower back stretch is one of the simplest stretching exercises to perform correctly without much instruction. It has great benefits for alleviating or preventing lower back pain, especially when combined with abdominal strengthening.

Walking is the simplest form of aerobic exercise. You can do it at a fitness center or on a treadmill at home if you choose, but more importantly, it can start and end at your own front door. No financial investment is necessary, and no special equipment is necessary, except for a good pair of walking shoes. Walking will provide a base of aerobic exercise on which you can build if you choose. After all, once you start walking, you may decide to go longer than 15 minutes. But you only need to go for 15 minutes to accomplish your goal. The additional exercises should only take an extra 5 minutes.

This is a great exercise program. Don't forget to congratulate yourself!

Tips for Getting Started

Before you begin, it's a good idea to decide the usual days and times on which you are going to do your new exercise routine. If you leave it vague as to which days of the week you'll exercise, it often doesn't happen. If you say to yourself, "I'll do my routine every Monday, Wednesday, and Saturday morning," you'll stand a better chance of doing it consistently. Actually, write it into your schedule. Even better! Sure, you'll switch days or times on occasion, but that'll be the exception, rather than the norm.

CARDIOVASCULAR EXERCISE – LEVEL 2
NEVER TOO EARLY

Walking is the simplest method to implement for cardiovascular exercise since you don't need to go to a special place or have access to special equipment. However, if you have access and enjoy something different, feel free to substitute a treadmill, elliptical machine, swimming, deep water running, or any other cardiovascular exercise. The only requirement is that you keep moving at a moderate level for 15 minutes.

NEVER TOO LATE

The cardiovascular component for this level is to simply walk for 15 minutes. One consideration may be weather or uneven surfaces. To reduce your risk of a fall, be careful of slippery conditions, such as rain or wet leaves, and only use a treadmill if your balance is good.

Aquatic exercise can be a great alternative if you have arthritis or other joint problems. Try water walking, shallow water aerobics, or deep water running with a floatation belt. All three will feel great on your joints while you get a great workout. If you have access to a fitness center, especially one that is specialized for older adults, you may find a seated elliptical machine, recumbent stationary bicycle, or a NuStep® machine, which are often comfortable for those with joint problems. Again, the only requirement is that you keep moving at a moderate level for 15 minutes.

Fitness Walking Tips

Since walking is the core aerobic exercise component for Level 2 for both NEVER TOO EARLY and NEVER TOO LATE, let's review some helpful walking tips.

Start and End at a Comfortable Pace
Be sure to warm-up and cool-down by simply walking at a slower pace during the first and last few minutes of your walk. The warm-up gradually prepares your body for exercise and the cool-down gradually brings your heart rate back to normal.

Watch Your Intensity
The goal intensity in exercise walking is a brisk pace. It shouldn't feel like a stroll, but it also shouldn't feel "really hard" either. A moderate, "somewhat hard" pace is the goal—one you can maintain for at least 15 minutes. The "Talk Test" is a good measure of intensity if you don't want to bother with the other methods outlined in Chapter Five. If you can't talk while walking, you're working too hard. If you can sing or talk at great length, you're probably not working hard enough!

Measure a Course...Or Not
Some people prefer to walk at a nearby track or on a measured route in order to determine how far they walk. Others prefer the simplicity of just starting and ending at their own front door. The choice is yours!

Keep It Up
Make walking a part of your daily activities. Put it on your schedule. Pick a time that is best for you. Enlist a friend to be a walking partner. Go to the mall on bad weather days. Vary the course to make it interesting. Consistency is always the goal!

When You're Ready for a Bigger Challenge
If you've been at it for a while and would like to step things up a notch, try adding some hills into your course or try "interval walking". With intervals, you sprinkle short bursts of a faster pace into your regular walk. These bursts can be one minute long or even less. They don't have to be structured, either. You may want to challenge yourself to "walk as fast as you can" to the next tree and then bring it back to your normal pace. A few minutes later, you may repeat the challenge.

How to Walk
It may sound odd to need instruction on "how" to walk. But when you're walking for exercise, it's helpful to know about correct posture, arm swing, and stride length.

Posture

Your whole body should lean slightly forward from the ankles. (Don't lean from the waist. This will make your back tired and breathing more difficult.) Keep your head and chin up, shoulders relaxed and pulled back, and your abdominal muscles tightened for good back support. (Sounds like a lot to think about? Try thinking about one or two tips at a time.)

Arm Swing

Try to keep your elbows bent at about a 90-degree angle or whatever is most comfortable for you. Swing from the shoulder, not the elbow. Your hands should not swing higher than chest level during the forward swing. Keep your arms close to your body and parallel to your body. If you use the 90-degree arm swing, you will burn 5–10% more calories than by just allowing your arms to swing naturally without thinking about it. However, it's not for everyone. You may feel awkward doing so, or just prefer not to. That's fine!

Stride

Avoid the tendency to take longer strides to go faster. Unlike runners, walkers need to move their feet faster by taking more steps per minute while maintaining their natural stride. With each step, your heel should strike the ground first, then roll through the ball of your foot and push off from the toe.

A Quick Stretch at the End

A quick calf stretch at the end of your walk is a good idea, especially if your pace is brisk. It's not the end of the world if you skip it, but read the following so at least you'll know what it is, should you choose to add it in:

Standing Calf Stretch

Stand with your feet together and take a big step backward with one foot. Next, shift your weight forward so that your front knee is bent, but the knee is not jutting out past your toes. Be sure to keep the heel of your back foot on the floor. If you don't feel a stretch in the calf of your back leg, you'll need to take a bigger step backwards with the back leg. Hold this position for about 15 seconds and then switch.

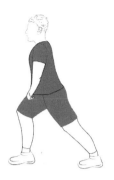

ABDOMINAL STRENGTHENING EXERCISE – LEVEL 2

NEVER TOO EARLY

Plank

Start on the floor lying on your stomach. Come up on your toes and forearms, keeping your body completely straight (don't let your hips sag down or pike up). If you find that this position is too intense, you can do the modified version on your toes and hands. The goal is to stay in this position for as long as possible. At first, this could be just ten seconds, but you will want to build up to 60 seconds or more. Once you are able to plank for more than a minute, you may be ready for more advanced abdominal strengthening exercises. This exercise should look familiar from the chapter on preventing back pain.

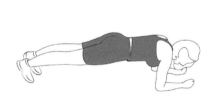
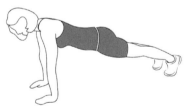

NEVER TOO LATE

Seated Abdominal Crunch

This abdominal exercise is ideal if you are not comfortable getting on the floor. In the starting position, you are sitting at the edge of the chair. Slowly lean back until you almost touch your shoulder blades to the back of the chair. You should feel your abdominal muscles tighten. Then slowly come back up to the starting position. Perform 5–20 repetitions as comfortable. This is the same exercise used in Chapter 9 on preventing back pain.

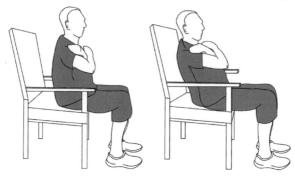

UPPER BODY STRENGTHENING EXERCISE – LEVEL 2
NEVER TOO EARLY

Push-ups

Start face down on your hands and knees or hands and feet. Be sure to keep your body rigid as you go down and up and focus on bending your elbows fully. Quite often, when you aren't quite strong enough to do the full range of motion correctly, your body will decide on its own to "cheat" 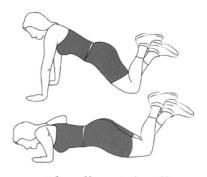 by not letting you go down very far or not bending at the elbow. (Your body is very wise—it doesn't want you to fall on your face!). Take that as an indicator to start with a less intense version that you can perform correctly and gradually build from there. The photo above shows "modified push-ups" on your knees. If the "modified" push up is too difficult, try "wall push-ups" by standing a few feet from a wall. Place your hands on the wall at shoulder height, bend your elbows and move your body towards and then away from the wall. If the modified version is too easy, you can do full body pushups on your toes with a straight body, but only if you can bend your elbows fully and keep your body straight while you lower completely to the floor and push back up. If an honest assessment shows that your rear end stays up while your head goes down, or you are sagging through the hips while trying to do a full body push-up, you're better off doing the modified push-up until you become stronger.

Never Too Late

Seated Press Ups

Start off seated with your hands on the arms of the chair and your feet flat on the floor. Press up on your hands until your elbows are straight. Do not use your legs to help. You will not end up standing up fully. Bend your elbows to lower your body back to the chair. Perform 5-20 repetitions as comfortable.

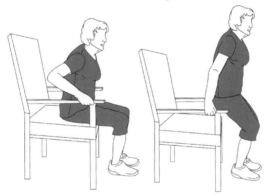

LOWER BODY STRENGTHENING EXERCISE – LEVEL 2

Never Too Early

Stationary Lunges

Stand in a wide lunge position with your feet parallel. The front foot is planted, and the back heel is raised up so your weight is on the ball of the foot only. Slowly lower your body down until your back knee almost touches the floor while letting your front knee bend to 90 degrees. Notice how your front knee stays straight above your front foot and does not push forward. Also notice how your body stays vertical from your head to your back knee. Push straight up through the heel of your front foot and the ball of your back foot until you are up again. Do not push

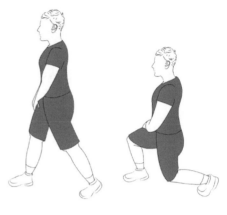

forward, only push up. Repeat the movement up to 10 or 20 times on one side before switching to the opposite foot in front.

Never Too Late

The Sit-to-Stand or Leg Extension

The Sit-to-Stand

Begin by sitting close to the end of the chair. The movement is quite straightforward: stand up and sit back down without using your arms to assist. This is the same exercise used in Chapter 9 for falls prevention.

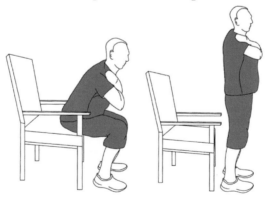

A few tips for doing this exercise:
  • Make sure the chair is sturdy (no wheels and not a flimsy chair). Push the chair up against a wall for maximum stability.

- How many? To test yourself, see how many you can do in 30 seconds.
  - If you are unable to do even one repetition, it would be unsafe to proceed, but that's ok! You can start with using your hands a bit and progress to removing them. If even that is too difficult, for safety, you will need to use the alternate exercise "leg extension" with the goal of building up your strength to the point that you can try the sit-to-stand again.
  - If you can do less than 10 repetitions, start with whatever amount you can do and then gradually build up to 10-20 or more. If you need a little help from your upper body to push off the chair or hold onto a railing, that's ok in the beginning, but the goal is to gradually be able to perform the exercise unassisted. You will get there if you do the exercise consistently!
  - If you can do 10 or more repetitions, continue to do as many as you can daily to maintain and build your strength. If you can do 30 or more, consider contacting a fitness professional for a more challenging exercise routine.

The Leg Extension

The Leg Extension is for you if you are unable to perform the sit-to-stand for even one repetition. Sit upright in a chair and lift one leg so that the knee is a bit higher than the other leg. Kick out your foot until your knee is straight, and then bend it to return to the starting position. If you don't keep your moving knee a bit higher than the stationary knee, your foot will bump into the floor and stop your range of motion before you fully return to the starting position. Perform 8–12 repetitions for each leg.

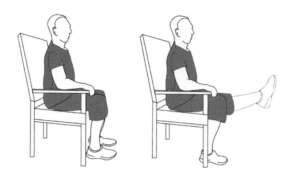

STRETCHING EXERCISE – LOWER BACK STRETCH – LEVEL 2

NEVER TOO EARLY

Lying, Knees to Chest

Lie on your back and pull both knees to your chest with your hands, clasping your hands under your knees if possible. Hold this position for at least 30 seconds, or as long as several minutes

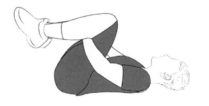

if you have chronic lower back pain. If you can only hold it for 30 seconds, repeat it several times. This should also look familiar from the chapter on preventing back pain.

NEVER TOO LATE

Lower Back Stretch—two choices

1. Seated Lower Back Stretch with Rounded Spine

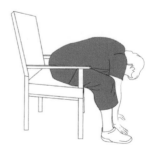

This is one of the gentlest varieties of a lower back stretch because you are seated, but it is *only* appropriate if you do not have osteoporosis. While seated, simply place your feet shoulder-width apart, round your back over, and let your head and hands lower down. Stay in this position for 15–30 seconds. Your lower back muscles will relax and lengthen.

2. *Seated Lower Back Stretch with a Straight Spine*

If you have osteoporosis, lean forward with a *straight* spine while keeping your hands on your thighs and do not lower your head below your knees. These are the same stretches featured in Chapter 9 for preventing back pain.

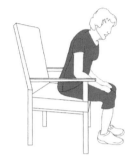

Whether it's **NEVER TOO EARLY** or **NEVER TOO LATE**, the Level 2: 20-minute no equipment home exercise plan is a great way to enjoy a fit lifestyle!

CHAPTER 13
LEVEL 3:
40-MINUTE MINIMAL EQUIPMENT
EXERCISE PLAN

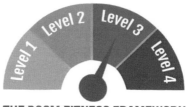

THE BOOM FITNESS FRAMEWORK

THE LEVEL 3: 40-Minute Minimal Equipment Exercise Plan is my favorite exercise level. It delivers great benefits, but is still realistic for many people's schedule. You'll need to plan for 40 minutes of intentional exercise, 3-4 times per week. Your Level 3 workout will include:

- 20 minutes of any cardiovascular exercise, 3–4 times per week (walking, jogging, elliptical machine, or stationary bicycle)

- A short (<20-minute) strength training routine, 3 times per week (one set of one exercise per muscle group)

- Several stretching exercises for key muscle groups

Did you notice that the 40-Minute Plan lists cardiovascular activity 3–4 times per week and strength training 3 times per week? The fourth cardiovascular/aerobic session is a "bonus"—if you can do it, great! You'll reap even more benefits. But if not, that's fine, too. Many people will prefer to schedule themselves three 40-minute time slots per week to do both their aerobic activity and their strength training together. If it's easier on your schedule, you can break them up. You will need a few inexpensive pieces of fitness equipment to perform the exercises for level 3. Visit www.CathyRichards.net/BoomExtras for more information on how to select and purchase exercise tubing, bands, and balls.

Let's look at the specifics for each of these components:

CARDIOVASCULAR EXERCISE – LEVEL 3

The Level 3 plan differs from Level 2 by upgrading from 15 to 20 minutes for your aerobic workout. This gets you into the gold standard "20 minutes or more" recommendations by the American College of Sports Medicine for cardiovascular exercise. (Less than 20 minutes still has value!)

NEVER TOO EARLY

Good choices include:

- Brisk walking (on a treadmill or outside)
  What's "brisk" for you will be subjective. Remember the intensity measures covered previously.

- Jogging (on a treadmill or outside)
  Jogging may be too intense for you, depending on your current fitness level. You would find this out if you tried to jog and needed to stop after just a few minutes. You might start with 4 or 5 minutes of walking for each 1 minute of jogging. Little by little, increase the amount of time you spend jogging and decrease the amount of time you spend walking. Make sure it's gradual and fun, if you choose to do so.

- Aquatic workouts such as swimming, deep water running, or aqua aerobics.

- Any aerobic exercise equipment that you find at a fitness center or that you can buy for home use:
  - Elliptical machine
  - Stationary bicycle
  - Cross country ski machine
- A dance aerobics class such as Zumba, or any other class listed as "cardio".

NEVER TOO LATE

The same cautions exist for cardiovascular exercise as with the Level 2. Walking is still a great choice, as are non-impact options such as aquatic exercise, a seated elliptical machine, recumbent stationary bicycle, or a NuStep® machine. Feel free to choose from other options listed on the "NEVER TOO EARLY" list if the movement is comfortable for your body and does not feel too intense to be able to continue for 20 minutes.

STRENGTH TRAINING ROUTINE – LEVEL 3

NEVER TOO EARLY (the NEVER TOO LATE routine begins on page 124)

As a starting point, this routine is designed as something that you can do at home. If you join a fitness center of some kind, your options for how to work each muscle group increase. At that point, you'll begin thinking in terms of working each muscle group, rather than following a list of exercises. You'll slowly learn several exercises for each muscle group and can begin to vary which exercise you do for each muscle group. For now, you will need to invest in a few pieces of inexpensive exercise equipment. You can find everything in the fitness section of many large retail stores, sporting goods store, or online.

Here's your shopping list:
- Two or Three Pairs of Dumbbells
- Exercise Tubing with Handles
- A Stability Ball (large, lightweight, inflated exercise ball)

You'll need two or three pairs of **dumbbells** because you'll be able to handle more weight for exercises that target larger muscle groups, while needing smaller weights for exercises that target smaller muscle groups. Remember from the chapter on resistance training that for each exercise you need a weight that causes you to reach fatigue between 8–15 repetitions.

Some people make the mistake of using dumbbells that are too light. One and 2-pound dumbbells are generally only appropriate for very frail individuals. They are often used in rehabilitation settings. It's more common for women to use anywhere from 3- to 15-pound dumbbells. For men, it is common to use from 10- to 30-pound dumbbells or even higher depending on your strength. Keep in mind that as your strength increases, you'll graduate to larger dumbbells over time. An ideal situation would be to try out each exercise with different size dumbbells before you buy them so that you know what weights you'll need.

Dumbbells are great for many exercises, but not all. Since dumbbells give you resistance against gravity, they only work as intended when pushing or pulling up a *vertical* plane. **Exercise tubing** is ideal for creating resistance in a *horizontal* plane or pulling *down*. It's also inexpensive, versatile, and perfect for travel. Both exercise tubing and bands comes in a variety of thicknesses that are usually color-coded—the thicker the tubing, the harder the resistance. Exercise bands can also accomplish the same thing. What's the difference between tubing and bands? Exercise tubing is easier to grip because of the handles, especially when using higher levels of resistance. This makes tubing just a bit more expensive. Exercise bands are large flat ribbons of elastic that work the same as tubing but are less expensive because they lack the handles. They are often sold in bulk rolls that are cut to be used in group settings but you can also find them sold individually.

Exercise balls known as "**stability balls**" are available in several sizes that correspond to your height. The most common ball sizes are "45 cm", "55 cm" and "65 cm". As a general guideline, if your height is less than 5'1", you will likely prefer a 45 cm ball. If your height is between 5'2"–5'8", a 55 cm ball. If you are over 5'9", a 65 cm ball. They are versatile, inexpensive, and fun to use.

You'll perform one set of each of the following ten exercises.

1. Dumbbell Chest Press (chest)

If you are using a bench, lie on your back. If you are using an exercise ball, sit on it and then walk your feet out until you are lying on the ball as pictured. Extend your arms up directly over your chest, with your elbows straight. Slowly bring your elbows down until the inside end of each dumbbell is touching the outside of your chest/armpit area. Bring the dumbbells back up to the starting position, keeping the dumbbells straight up over your chest (don't let them drift over your face or stomach).

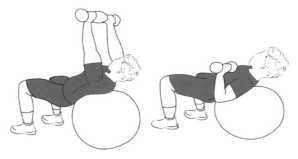

2. Seated Tubing Row (back)

Sit on the floor with your feet wider than shoulder width apart and your knees slightly bent. Wrap the tubing around the instep portion of both shoes. (Don't try this barefoot—ouch!) Criss-cross the tubing, forming an "X", and then hold the tubing itself, as opposed to the handles. (When you hold the handles, unless you have very long arms, you'll likely

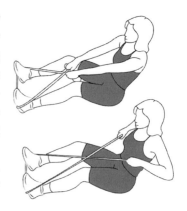

find there is too much slack in the tubing, making the exercise too easy.) Pull your elbows back, being conscious to squeeze your shoulder blades together. Slowly return to the starting position.

3. Dumbbell Side Raise (shoulders)

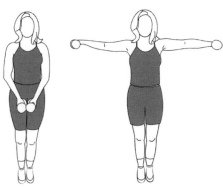

Stand, holding dumbbells in front of your body, palms facing each other. Slowly lift your arms up to the side until they are horizontal, keeping your elbows slightly bent. Your wrists should remain straight. When you get to the top, your wrists and elbows should be the same height, with your palms facing the floor. Slowly lower down to the starting position. If the dumbbells are too heavy, you won't be able to keep your elbows and wrists level, nor your palms facing down. You also want to avoid arching your back, which can happen if the dumbbells are too heavy. Think of the ending position as that of a male gymnast in the rings or imagine yourself holding a bucket in each hand. If your arms twist so that your palms no longer face the floor, you will spill your buckets of water.

4. Dumbbell Bicep Curl (biceps)

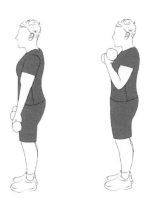

Begin with your arms at your sides with your palms facing front. Begin bending one elbow, so that when you end, your palm is facing your chest in front. Return to starting position and then begin the other arm. To make it more challenging (and finish more quickly), you can do both arms at the same time. Regardless, be sure that your elbows always go from completely straight to completely bent and don't use momentum to swing the dumbbell up. When you lower your arm down, the temptation is to stop and start coming back up before your elbow is completely straight. That's the easy way out! Keep yourself honest by going all the way down and all the way up. If you can't go all the way down before coming back up or you start arching your back, the weight is probably too heavy.

5. Dumbbell Overhead Triceps Extension (triceps)

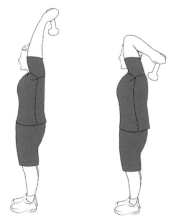

Hold one dumbbell overhead, as pictured. Notice that you are not holding the middle of the dumbbell, but rather, you slip the middle part between your thumb and index finger of both hands, and then grip the end of the dumbbell. Keep your elbows close to your head. Slowly bend your elbows so that the dumbbell drops low behind your head. Then, straighten your elbows again to return the dumbbell to the starting position. (When returning to the starting position, be sure that you are not moving your shoulder joints, which would throw the entire movement forward. Only move your elbow joints.)

6. Squats: Ball Squat or Dumbbell Squat (quadriceps and gluteus maximus)

The squat is one of my favorite exercises. It's a great way to work both your thighs and rear end at the same time. The ball squat is great for beginners because it is less intense and easier to perform correctly since the ball guides you through the correct range of motion. Dumbbell squats are more advanced, requiring more effort to maintain the proper form. Pay careful attention to the instructions below because performing squats incorrectly can put your knees at risk for injury. Try the ball squat first and if it's too easy, move on to the dumbbell squat.

The Ball Squat

Find a wall surface that is flat and bare (no door-knobs, light switches, or picture frames). Place the ball between you and the wall, about waist height and then put your back to the ball. Press the small of your back firmly against the ball. It should feel like 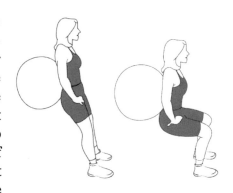 the ball "fits" comfortably in the arch of your back. Adjust your feet so that they are about shoulder-width apart and parallel to each other. Make sure your feet are also several feet away from the wall. If your feet are too close to the wall, your knees will jut out uncomfortably once you begin the motion. If this happens to you, move your feet a few more inches away from the wall and try again. It may take a few tries to find the right foot placement for you based on your height.

The Motion

Slowly begin squatting down by bending your knees and curling your tailbone under the ball until your thighs are almost parallel to the floor (approaching a 90-degree bend at the knee joint). Your lower leg should remain fairly vertical, which keeps your knees over your ankles, not jutting out past your toes. Focus on keeping contact with the ball and avoid leaning forward. Once you reach the bottom of the range of motion, push straight up to your starting position. The ball should roll with you right back to its starting position at the small of your back.

How Far Down?

Knowing how far down to go is important and may take some practice. For some people, going all the way down to the point that their thighs are parallel to the floor, is uncomfortable. You may only go half that distance and that's okay. You may find that as you build strength, you can gradually go further down. Pay attention to what your knees are telling you and only perform the exercise through the range of motion that is comfortable for you. (Note to overachievers: "Parallel" is the most advanced stopping point. It is never advisable to go past the parallel point, as that is stressful for your knee joints.)

Note: If the ball slips and starts to fall to the ground, you are performing the exercise incorrectly. Check to see if you are either leaning forward, not pressing the small of your back into the ball, and/or not curling your tailbone under the ball as you go down.

Dumbbell Squats

Stand with your feet slightly wider than shoulder-width apart. Brace the dumbbells on your shoulders as pictured. (Once you are experienced, you will probably use your heaviest dumbbells for this exercise. When you're just starting out, begin with light dumbbells or no weights at all until you get the hang of it.)

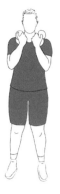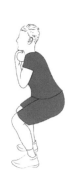

Slowly bend your knees and arch your back as you press your hips and butt out behind you. Try to keep your chest up. The goal is to lower down until your thighs are almost parallel to the floor without letting your knees jut out past your toes. This means that your ankle joints aren't bending at all. Once again, don't go past the parallel point. When you start coming back up, thrust your hips forward in a subtle way so that your body is straight once again.

A Few Words of Caution about Squats
Stop if you feel pain, especially in your knees. You may want to double check to make sure you are using the correct form. But even performed correctly, squats may not be for you. Listen to your body and if it hurts, don't do it.

7. Ball Hamstring Curl (hamstrings)

This is a fun exercise that may take a little practice at first in order to keep your balance. Lie on the floor on your back with your calves and ankles propped up on the ball. If the ball is too close to you (under your knees), you won't have enough room to let the ball roll. If the ball is too far away from you (under your ankles and feet only), it 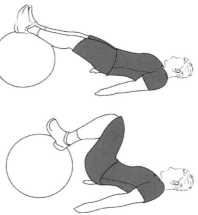 will probably slip away. Brace yourself with your arms pressing down on the floor and lift up your hips. (This is where you may need to practice your balance!) While keeping your hips elevated, dig your heels into the ball and roll the ball toward your rear end, then roll back out. You may need to occasionally reposition your feet if the ball starts slipping away from you.

8. Inner Thigh Ball Squeeze (adductors/inner thigh)

Approach the ball from behind and carefully sit on it. Roll forward slightly until your hip joint is completely straight. (Your knees are pointing down, not forward, and your feet are behind you.) If you fall off the front of the ball, try again but this time, start farther back. Once you're in a comfortable position, simply squeeze the ball with your thighs and release. I like to finish with an extended squeeze of 10 or more seconds.

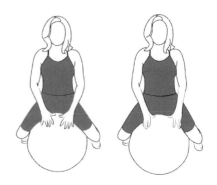

9. Lying Hip Abduction with Tubing (abductors/hips)

Lie on your back on the floor, with the tubing around your feet. Be sure that the tubing is securely caught in the notch of your shoe at the instep. Your legs are overhead, but angled down a bit (not straight up), and your knees are slightly bent. You'll want about 6-10 inches of tubing between your feet. If you

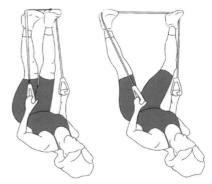

feel any cramping in your hip muscles, try angling your legs down even farther. Open and close your legs from the hip joint. Each time you press out, the tubing will stretch and apply a resistance to your hip muscles doing the work. Press out and release back in as many times as you can.

10. Plank (abdominals)

Start on the floor lying on your stomach. Come up on your toes and forearms, keeping your body completely straight (don't let your hips sag down or pike up). If you find that this position is too intense, you can do the modified version on your toes and hands. The goal is to stay in this position for as long as possible. At first, this could be just ten seconds, but you will want to build up to sixty seconds or more. Once you are able to plank for more than a minute, you may be ready for more advanced abdominal strengthening exercises. This exercise should look familiar from the chapter on preventing back pain and also from Level 2.

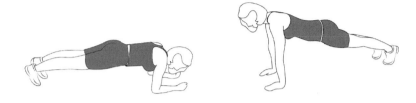

Caution

Not all exercises are suitable for all people. Please check with your physician before starting this or any exercise routine. If a particular exercise is painful for you, please skip it. It's always wise to warm-up with light movement for 3-5 minutes before beginning.

This top-ten list allows you to work every major muscle group in twenty minutes or less. Can you start with just a few and build up to all ten later? Absolutely. Can you skip a muscle group or two when you are short on time? Absolutely! Remember, more may be better than less, but some is better than none. Balance, proper form, and posture are important in doing each exercise correctly—both for maximum benefit and for injury prevention. You'll be performing one set of 8–15 repetitions for all of the dumbbell exercises. With ball or tubing exercises, it's more difficult to increase the resistance, therefore, depending on your strength, you'll just do more repetitions until you reach fatigue—it could be as many as 30–50 repetitions.

If you plan on using exercise tubing, note that when you purchase the tubing, it is color-coded for thickness/intensity. When one color is too easy, you can purchase a thicker tube. You probably remember from our chapter on strength training that performing high reps with a limited resistance isn't ideal for strength gains, but it's the best we have available for exercise tubing. You'll still get plenty of good results as long as you continue until your muscles feel fatigued. Don't stop the minute it starts to feel difficult!

NEVER TOO EARLY Stretching Exercises begin on page 130.

NEVER TOO LATE

For older adults, stronger muscles mean being able to carry your own groceries, get out of a chair with ease, and walk farther and faster. Stronger muscles help ward off joint problems, decrease the risk of osteoporosis, and improve posture and back pain. Remember that research shows that the human body responds to strength training well into advanced age. Since the Level 3 program includes more than a few exercises, this is a good time to review some of the physical changes that are common as we age and that we are addressing in this exercise routine. Good for us that exercise can improve all of these items.

- The shoulders of older adults can often be a bit rounded and asymmetrical in height. This makes posture exercises and stretching for the chest and front of the shoulders beneficial. Start right now. Pull your shoulders back and squeeze your shoulder blades together. Feel better? Take note of the chest stretch shown later in this chapter also.

- It's common as we age for our head to sit a bit more forward than it should. Try pulling your chin in and also stretching and strengthening the neck muscles.

- The range of motion and strength for knee flexion and extension (bending and straightening) may be reduced, accompanied by weakness of the hip abductors (ability to lift your leg out to the side) and ankle dorsiflexors (ability to pull your toes up toward your shin). The Achilles tendon often shortens as well. Ankle circles, and pointing-flexing your toes are all great for you. Go ahead and stand up and lift and lower your leg to the side while standing and then bend and straighten your knee.

- Range of motion in the pelvis can be reduced a bit. Try doing the motion of a hula hoop slowly. It should feel great!

- Having strong calf muscles is important for balance and walking gait, so including calf stretching and strengthening is valuable.

- If you have osteoporosis, your doctor has likely warned you to only bend forward a small amount. Do not do any exercises that cause you to bend over completely.

- If you have arthritis, you will have some days that your joints feel better than others. Daily range of motion exercises are helpful, but only through the range that is comfortable. On flair-up days, you will want to do less, but try to do more on other days. I've heard it said that exercise can be uncomfortable with arthritis, but if you don't exercise, you will be more uncomfortable all the time.

You will need: An Exercise Band

From the comfort of a chair and using an exercise band, the exercise routine that follows can build substantial strength. Exercise bands are easy to use, inexpensive, versatile, and come in a variety of resistance levels. You can also use exercise tubing with handles, but the bands tend to be easier to keep in place during each exercise.

A few overall guidelines:

- Make sure the chair you have selected is sturdy and does not have wheels.

- Perform each exercise slowly and smoothly.

- For each exercise, move through the full range of motion as much as possible as long as no pain is experienced.

- Breathe evenly during the full range of motion. Do not hold your breath during any portion of the exercise.

- Perform approximately 8–15 repetitions of each exercise or until you feel as though the muscles are fatigued and you can't comfortably do any more. Feeling fatigued is different than feeling pain.

- The amount of resistance used will impact how quickly the muscles feel fatigued. With exercise bands, this means considering how much or how little slack you have in the band based on where you grip the band. Adjust

your grip until the exercise feels somewhat challenging—
not too hard, nor too easy.

- If you experience true pain, especially in a joint, stop
immediately.

1. Seated Chest Press

Wrap the exercise band behind your back and grip it on each side
under your armpits. Press out in front of you until your elbows are
almost straight. Slowly return to starting position and repeat.

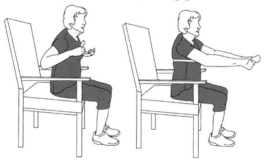

2. Seated Row

Sit upright close to the edge of the chair with your legs extended
a bit, heels anchored to the floor, and knees slightly bent. Wrap
the exercise band around your feet, crisscross the band, and then
hold one end in each hand. (Be sure that the band is anchored
securely around the instep of your shoe. Do not let the band slide
up towards your toes as it could slip off and ricochet towards
your face!) Pull on the band, squeezing your shoulder blades
together. Slowly return to starting position and repeat.

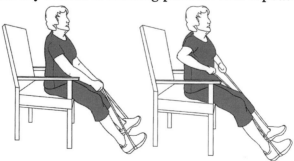

3. Biceps Curl

Sit with feet firmly planted on the floor in front of you. Anchor the band securely under your feet and grip firmly with each hand. Keeping your elbows by your side, bend your elbows ending with your palms near your shoulders. Slowly return to starting position and repeat.

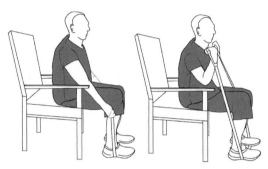

4. Triceps Extension

Grip the band with both hands in front of you, leaving 8-12 inches of band between your hands. Anchor one hand right above your chest. With the other arm, extend the elbow until your arm is straight out to the side. Slowly return to starting position and repeat.

5. Seated Abdominal Crunch

Sit upright close to the edge of the chair and cross your arms over your chest. Slowly lean back until your shoulder blades barely touch the back of the chair. Hold for just a moment, then slowly return to the starting position and repeat.

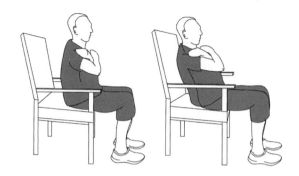

6. Leg Press

Sitting upright, lift one leg, wrap the band around the bottom of your shoe, and grip firmly in each hand. Press your foot out until the knee is almost straight. Slowly return to starting position and repeat. Switch to the other leg.

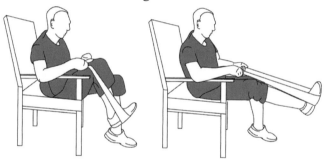

7. Ankle Circles and Point/Flex

While seated, extend one leg out and slowly circle your ankle joint, creating as big of a range of motion as possible with your toes. Do several revolutions in each direction. Then point and flex your ankle by pulling your toes firmly toward your shin and then pointing your toes away from you as firmly as possible. Repeat several times.

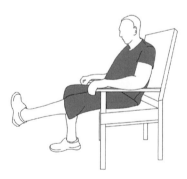

8. Side Leg Lift

Standing at a wall or holding on to a chair, lift your leg out to the side. Keep your posture straight and do not lean over to the opposite side as you lift the leg. You should only be able to lift it a small amount. Lower the leg, but do not let it touch the floor before lifting again, unless you really need to!

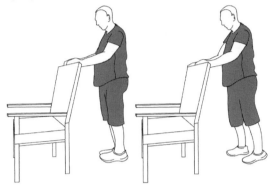

9. Standing Calf Raise

Stand on both feet at a wall or holding on to a chair. Slowly rise up on your toes and then lower back down. For a higher intensity version and if your balance is very good, stand on one foot with the non-weight bearing foot propped behind the other ankle. If performing the one-leg version, you will need to switch to the other leg when you are done.

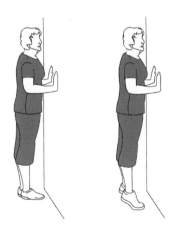

10. Chin Tuck

Seated or standing, pull your chin back towards you and hold for 5-10 seconds. Repeat. When you release, try not to release fully to the point that your head started at, as we all tend to carry our head too far forward, which throws our body alignment off.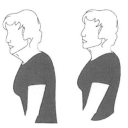

Strength training is for everybody. The benefits will add up for years to come!

NEVER TOO LATE Stretching Exercises begin on page 131.

STRETCHING EXERCISES – LEVEL 3
NEVER TOO EARLY

Four Key Stretches

A great way to finish off your Level 3 exercise routine is with a few stretches for the major muscle groups most in need of some TLC after a workout. You can hold each stretch for as little as 10–15 seconds for a quick stretch, up to 30 seconds when you're relaxing a little more into the stretch, or as long as a full minute when you are nursing a problem in that area. Remember not to bounce.

1. Quadriceps Stretch

Stand on one foot and hold the other foot up behind you as pictured. Be sure to keep your knees close together.

2. Chest Stretch

Let your arms fall open wide. Pull your arms back, squeezing your shoulder blades together.

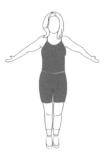

3. Lower Back Stretch

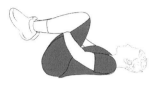

Lie on your back and pull both knees into your chest, clasping your hands under your knees if possible. Hold this position for at least 30 seconds, or as long as several minutes if you have chronic lower back pain. If you can only hold it for 30 seconds, repeat it several times. This should also look familiar from the chapter on preventing back pain and Level 2.

4. Hamstring Stretch

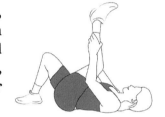

While lying on the floor on your back, keep one leg bent with your foot flat on the floor. Extend the other leg up and pull towards your body with your hands, keeping your knee slightly bent and your lower back pressed to the floor. Switch.

NEVER TOO LATE

Four Key Stretches

There are four different stretches for **Level 3 NEVER TOO LATE**. You can hold each stretch for as little as 10–15 seconds for a quick stretch, or up to 30 seconds when you're relaxing a little more into the stretch. Remember to ease into the stretch and not to bounce.

1. Seated Chest Stretch

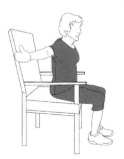

Let your arms fall open wide. Pull your arms back, squeezing your shoulder blades together.

2. Seated Lower Back Stretch

While seated close to the end of the chair, place your feet shoulder-width apart, round your back over, and let your head and hands lower down. If you have osteoporosis, lean forward with a *straight* spine while keeping your hands on your thighs and do not lower your head below your knees.

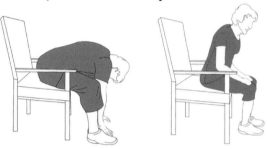

3. Seated Hamstring Stretch

Sit close to the end of the chair with one leg straight out in front of you on your heel. Gently lean forward towards the straight leg.

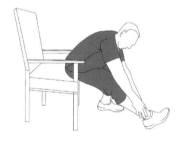

4. Neck Stretch

Seated or standing, gently tilt your ear towards your shoulder. To deepen the stretch, you can gently pull on your head and also extend the opposite arm out to the side. Switch.

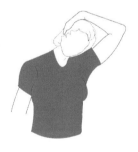

The Level 3 40-Minute Minimal Equipment Exercise Plan is a great way to live a fit lifestyle!

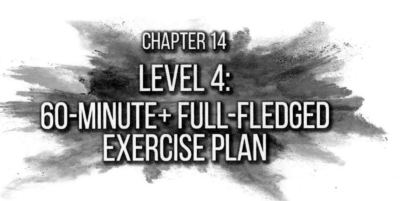

CHAPTER 14
LEVEL 4:
60-MINUTE+ FULL-FLEDGED
EXERCISE PLAN

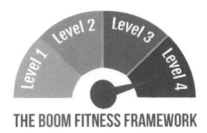

THE BOOM FITNESS FRAMEWORK

THE LEVEL 4: 60-Minute+ Full-Fledged Exercise Plan involves the highest level of time commitment and is reserved for those who really enjoy exercise, have ambitious goals, or both! You'll need to plan for more than 60 total minutes of intentional exercise, 3-6 times per week. (The 60 minutes doesn't have to be done all at once.) Your Level 4 workout will include:

- 20–60 minutes of any aerobic exercise, 3–5 times per week (walking, jogging, dance aerobics, elliptical machine, or stationary bicycle)
- A 30–40-minute strength training routine, 3 times per week (2–3 sets per muscle group)
- Stretching exercises for each major muscle group, 3 or more times per week

CARDIOVASCULAR EXERCISE — LEVEL 4
NEVER TOO EARLY AND NEVER TOO LATE

Once you are invested enough in a fit lifestyle to be interested in a Level 4 program, you will likely want to mix up your modes and lengths of your cardiovascular workouts. The recommended forms of exercise are the same as for Level 3. The only difference is the number of days per week and the length of the workouts. Seek the assistance of a fitness professional to ensure that you aren't overdoing it.

STRENGTH TRAINING AND STRETCHING — LEVEL 4
NEVER TOO EARLY AND NEVER TOO LATE

A Level 4 program involves an increase in intensity by performing more sets per muscle group in the strength training routine and also including a stretch for each major muscle group. When you are doing more than one set per muscle group, the strength training principles that were outlined in Chapter 6 become very important. As with your cardiovascular exercise, you will likely want to include some variety in the exercises you choose from day to day. Again, the assistance of a fitness professional will be valuable to get the most out of your workouts and also to make sure you are using proper form to prevent injury.

The Level 4 plan is a comprehensive approach that will bring you many benefits!

STEP FOUR:

FUELING UP AND BALANCING THE SCALE

CHAPTER 15

FUELING UP FOR A STRONG BODY, SHARP BRAIN, AND ENDLESS ENERGY

"*E*AT A DONUT, *run like a donut.*" This is a funny old quote from a runner I knew when I was younger. For some reason, it has stuck with me all these years. You don't have to be a runner to get the gist. *"You are what you eat"* comes to mind as well.

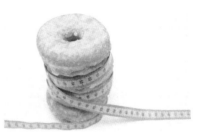

Eating healthier doesn't mean we have to give up all our favorite foods and resign ourselves to eating rabbit food. Just as with exercise, even small changes can go a long way. For general good health, most of us know what foods we need to eat more and less of and we know that moderation is a key concept. Unfortunately, an "all or none" mindset can creep into our eating patterns as it does with exercise, and we know that it just doesn't work. A good rule of thumb is to stay away from fad diets and extremes of any kind and stick with the tried and true basics most of the time.

As with many things in life, the 80/20 rule is a good approach for healthy eating if you don't have a medical condition that requires vigilant monitoring. This means eating a mostly healthy diet 80% of the time, with the primary purpose of eating to *fuel* our body and our brain. The other 20% of the time, for special events or vacations, for instance, the primary purpose shifts to enjoyment and celebration. For these occasions, most of us can enjoy the foods of our choice without guilt. The problems crop up when the good times keep rolling and we don't know how to get back to a more reasonable eating plan after the special event, or when we choose unhealthy options on a day-in, day-out basis over many years.

Consistent with our overall theme, eating for a strong body, a sharp brain, and endless energy are all based on the *same* recommendations. The same foods that make our body stronger also make our brain sharper and give us more energy! We will focus on "eat more of" and "eat less of" instead of any specific recommendations. You will probably not see any surprises, but rather reinforcement for an eating style that you already know is good for you. As you review the lists to come, use a critical eye to pick out one or two small changes that seem reasonable to make and that you can see yourself still doing a year from now. Long term changes lead to long term results. Short term changes often lead to a rebound effect from overly restrictive efforts or a feeling of deprivation.

The recommendations outlined here are designed for general health and energy. If you have a specific medical condition that warrants a closely monitored diet, you could benefit from a consultation with a registered dietitian.

Things we need to eat MORE of:

- Natural, unprocessed foods
  Challenge yourself to focus your diet on foods that don't have a long list of unrecognizable ingredients and aren't wrapped in cellophane packaging.

- Whole grains
  Carbohydrates have gotten a bad name lately, but the whole grain variety serve a very important role in a healthy diet and are an important source of energy. Good examples include 100% whole grain breads and

cereals, pastas made with whole-wheat, and grains such as bulgur, cornmeal, oatmeal, and brown rice instead of white bread, regular pasta, and white rice.

- Fiber – 25 grams per day
  Fiber is one of the most important elements to keep yourself feeling full and to ensure that your digestive system works comfortably. This means lots of whole fruits and vegetables, whole grains, beans, and lentils. Read labels or use a food diary to get a feeling of how to get to 25 grams easily.

- Lean and plant-based proteins
  Aim to have a protein source with each meal. The best varieties include fish, lean poultry, beans, and lentils.

- Healthy fats
  Fat is not the enemy. We need a certain amount of healthy fats in our diet daily, such as those found in olive oil, nuts and avocado to keep us feeling full and help stabilize blood sugar levels. Let's be honest, though—not many people need to "try" to get more fat in their diet, so a better goal is to try to choose healthier fats. When we have too much overall fat in our diet or too much of the unhealthy kind, problems arise for heart health and weight gain. Fat should make up no more than 30% of our diet, which works out to be about 25-75 total grams of fat per day, depending on your total calories.

- Fruits and vegetables
  Eat every kind and any kind—the more the better! There is one exception—it's wise to limit fruit juices, which provide too much sugar in a concentrated form. Yes, it's "natural sugar" but it can still wreak havoc by adding unintentional calories and making your blood sugar level rise too quickly. Try making a sheet pan of roasted vegetables as often as possible—it's a super tasty way to get your veggies. All you need to do

is spread them out, drizzle with a little olive oil, and bake at 400 degrees for about 30 minutes, stirring occasionally.

- The "Superfoods"
  Check out this list! My version of superfoods meets *all* the previous recommendations. One benefit of eating more of the superfoods is that each time you choose a superfood, it's one less situation in which you are eating something *less* virtuous.

SUPERFOODS		
Tomatoes	Spinach	Yogurt
Broccoli	Whole Grains	Salmon
Sweet Potatoes	Edamame	Quinoa
Avocado	Winter Squashes	Barley
Pumpkin	Nuts and Seeds	Farro
Beans	Leafy greens	Berries
Lentils	Flax Seed	

Things we need to eat LESS of:

- White flour
  Pasta, rice, and breads that are made with white flour have less fiber and less nutrition. They will also leave you hungry sooner. Choose whole grain options as much as you can.

- Sugar
  We know this category well—sweets, pastries, and a whole lot more. Most of us eat a lot more sugar than we think. It's in oh, so many processed foods and colors our taste buds. Once you intentionally minimize the sugar in your diet, you will notice a huge difference in how you feel.

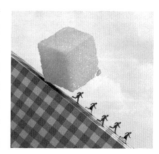

- Saturated and partially hydrogenated fat
Saturated fats are found in meat, dairy, and eggs. Limit fatty cuts of meat and full fat dairy options. Cheese is a favorite food of so many people, but the fat and calories can get out of hand quickly, so it's best to keep an eye on it. Eggs have had a controversial history in nutrition recommendations. Current research says that eggs, in moderation, can be part of a healthy diet. Partially hydrogenated fats are found in packaged goods and just about everything in the snack food aisle of the grocery store. It's best to just avoid that aisle as much as possible.

- Processed foods
This would be the opposite of "natural foods". These are items that come prepackaged, with long lists of ingredients that you can't pronounce. They are often high in sugar, fat, salt, and preservatives. Once again, you know which grocery aisles are filled with these items, so try to steer clear!

- Fried foods
Fried chicken, French fries, and deep-fried anything spell trouble. Fried foods go in the category of eating for pleasure on special occasions—if that. They have no business as a part of your everyday diet. Not only are vegetable oils processed poorly in the way they are heated up and broken down, but businesses that serve fried foods usually don't change their oil very frequently. If oil is reused over and over again it starts breaking down and oxidizing which releases free radicals and could increase your risk of cancer—yikes! There are alternatives that your taste buds can adapt to fairly easily. Let's take French fries – baked fries taste just as good as the deep-fried variety. Throw the freezer variety on a cookie sheet or cut your own and toss in olive oil and into the oven.

- Meat and dairy in general

  It is helpful to your health to choose lean meat and dairy vs. full-fat varieties most of the time. One step better is to eat less meat and dairy products overall. Try increasing your intake of fish and plant-based proteins by enjoying "Meatless Mondays" to experiment with vegetarian or vegan options. You won't feel good if you cut out meat and dairy without substituting other sources of protein, so experiment with beans, lentils, and more. You don't need to be fully vegan to gain the benefits. The phrase "plant-based diet" demonstrates a philosophy of moderation in this area, and trying to choose plants for your protein source more often than meat or dairy. Try it!

- Alcohol

  Despite some of the benefits that we hear about red wine, in general, alcohol has a negative effect on most health areas. Many people can enjoy it in moderation, however, keep in mind that alcohol dehydrates us and wreaks havoc on our brain cells and body weight without adding any nutritional value. Excessive use is linked to not only addiction, but a multitude of diseases including liver disease, cancer, heart disease, diabetes, and cognitive diseases. If you choose to partake in alcohol, be sure to consume it in moderation.

Other Healthy Eating Tips

Besides identifying what foods to eat more of and less of, there are other nutrition-related factors that help us achieve a strong body, sharp brain, and endless energy.

- Calorie Intake and Nutritional Value

  Obviously, total calories matter. Too few calories and you won't have enough energy. Too many calories and you'll end up overweight, which brings a host of its own problems. How do you know how many calories to eat in a day? For most people, it's not necessary to *count* calories, but an approximation can be helpful. There are general guidelines based on calculations using your body weight and goals. One of the best ways to get a customized range for you is through a free food tracking website such as www.MyFitnessPal.com. I am a big fan of food logging to get an eye-opening look at *exactly* what you are eating. Even if you don't think it's something you could do long term, you can gain an accurate picture of your typical diet by logging everything you eat for just a few days. I have seen more clients turn their diets around with information gleaned from a few days of food logging than any other tool.

- The Right Mix of Nutrients
  As with tracking calories, technology has made it much easier than in the past to know how much we need of different nutrients and match that information up with what we are actually eating. Once again, my go-to resource is www.MyFitnessPal.com. In addition to tracking your total calories, you will see targets and your totals of the specific nutrients you choose to track, starting with the basics of carbohydrates, protein, and fat, but then adding on additional values such as sugar, sodium, iron, calcium, or any other nutrient. Check it out!

- Spreading Out Your Calories
  A wise goal is to never be starving and never be stuffed. I don't know anyone who makes wise food choices when they are starving. Stuffed is no good either. Where do you think the body puts all those excess calories from a meal that it cannot digest in a reason-able amount of time? (You'd be

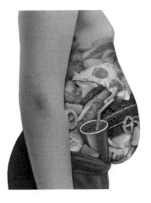

correct if you guessed your fat cells.) Try eating four to six times per day—mealtimes plus one or two healthy, pre-planned snacks. When you eat frequently, your blood sugar level will stay more even, which will decrease cravings. You will also be less likely to gain weight if you allow your body to take in calories little by little through the day as you burn them instead of overloading it with too many calories all at one time.

- Have a Little Protein or Fat with Each Meal or Snack
  Including protein or fat at every meal or snack will help slow down the digestive process and help you feel full longer. Carbohydrates are digested much more quickly when they are eaten alone, leading to a quicker turnaround time when you are hungry again.

- Stay Educated
  Check out one of my favorite resources—www.NutritionAction.com to stay up to date on interesting and realistic healthy eating tips. The website and newsletters are written with a no-nonsense approach and provide practical inform-ation you can implement today for healthier eating!

Never Too Early Fueling Up

Being on-the-go can be a slippery slope for your nutritional needs. Don't let a rushed lifestyle lead to poor habits.

Never Too Late Fueling Up

Ask your doctor if there are certain nutrients that you should be more concerned with than others. Be sure to stay well hydrated. Sometimes a reduced appetite makes it harder to get all the nutrients you need, so make your food choices count!

HYDRATION

While we focus on eating, let's not forget another important aspect of what we consume—what we *drink*. Hydration is vital for a strong body, sharp brain, and endless energy. Many people don't realize that dehydration is a significant source of fatigue. Water is also crucial for brain function and for our muscles.

You've probably heard that water comprises a significant percentage of an adult's body. We must replenish it, or we just won't feel good. Water is my favorite beverage.

Of course, fluid comes from some of our foods as well, but to ensure we have enough fluid, plain old everyday water is the BEST. A good challenge would be to get used to drinking straight water as your primary source of fluid. You will feel so much better and save on calories. Many people are not aware of how many calories they are consuming through beverages alone.

Another problem is when your consumption of caffeinated beverages dehydrates your body and causes you to need even more water to counteract the effect. The recommendations about exactly how much water we need continue to be vague. The eight glasses a day recommendation has been questioned, but we do know that by the time you feel thirsty, your body is probably already dehydrated. Proper hydration should lead to the urge to empty your bladder every few hours and your urine should be very pale in color. If you crave the carbonation of soda, a good alternative could be soda waters. Check out some on the market that take the oils from lemon or orange peel to add flavor naturally and without added sugar.

START EVERY DAY WITH A POWER BREAKFAST

Rule #1: Don't Skip It

It's not called "the most important meal of the day" for no reason. Let's start with the impact breakfast has on your metabolism.

Your body burns calories all day and all night, but your metabolism is at its slowest while you are asleep. The act of eating and digesting kick starts your metabolism, and therefore, it's important to have breakfast after eight hours at its slowest rate. Without breakfast, you'll be burning calories at a slower rate all the way up until you finally eat something. If you find that you are not waking up hungry, try having a smaller dinner. You might be in the habit of skipping breakfast because you are overeating at dinner. As mentioned earlier, it's much better to spread out your calories, and if there's a time of day to have more calories, a better choice would be in the morning instead of in the evening, when you will have a greater opportunity to burn them.

Rule #2: Avoid a "Carbohydrate Only" Breakfast… Especially If It's All Refined Sugar

Look at any "continental breakfast" and you'll see it: bagels, English muffins, donuts, muffins, coffee cakes, and to add insult to injury, fruit juices. It all seems harmless, but when you eat sugary refined carbohydrates for breakfast alone, they are digested very quickly and cause a quick increase in blood sugar. Your body responds with increased insulin production to buffer the sugar. Unfortunately, with such a quick and large surge of sugar, the insulin production often overshoots what is needed, with the result of *low* blood sugar not long after a sugary meal. That's why you end up feeling tired, sleepy, and hungry again soon after a carbohydrate-heavy meal. Even if you choose a healthy carbohydrate, such as a piece of fruit, pair it with a protein and/or fat to slow digestion and increase satiety. Try a pear with cheese, an apple with Greek yogurt, or a banana with peanut butter.

Rule #3: Seek a High Fiber and Protein Breakfast Choice

Carbohydrates are still the best energy source. The trick is to seek carbohydrates that are high in fiber—whole fruits instead of fruit juices, high fiber/low sugar breakfast cereals instead of sugary ones, and high fiber whole grain bread products instead of the processed, sugary, or fatty breads. The fiber slows down your digestion so that blood sugar increases more slowly and gradually. The result is a more modest insulin reaction and therefore no rebound low blood sugar. You'll feel full longer and all but abolish that gnawing "I'm still hungry, what else can I eat" feeling. Including protein with your breakfast has the same effect as the increased fiber: slowing down the digestion process, helping maintain a more stable blood sugar level that prevents food cravings, and feeling fuller for longer.

Rule #4: Don't Let the Protein Lead to Fatty Choices

By adding protein to your breakfast, steer clear of regular sausage, bacon, or excessive eggs and cheese. Whole eggs in moderation are fine for most people. Other low-fat protein choices for breakfast include turkey bacon, a sprinkling of low-fat cheese, skim or 1% milk, unsweetened almond milk, low-fat yogurt, or cottage cheese.

Putting It Together

What did you have for breakfast this morning? Was it Power Breakfast material? You've probably already guessed that toaster strudel and your local drive-thru don't fit the bill, but some others might surprise you.

What the Power Breakfast *ISN'T*

- The sausage-egg-cheese biscuit routine will leave you feeling fatty.
- The kids' sugar cereal with a glass of OJ will leave you feeling sugar shocked.
- Most average, non-sugary breakfast cereals will leave you feeling empty. Even if they're not too high in sugar, you'll still end up feeling hungry a short time after breakfast because they lack adequate fiber and protein to keep you feeling full.

What the Power Breakfast *IS*

A power breakfast is the kind of breakfast that leaves you feeling full, satisfied, and ready to start your day, and it keeps you feeling satisfied for at least three hours after breakfast. It doesn't leave you craving more sugary foods and it doesn't leave you hungry again soon after breakfast. Remember that in order to qualify as a power breakfast, your choice needs to have the following criteria:

- Low Sugar
- Low Fat
- High Protein
- High Fiber
- Lots of vitamins and minerals as an extra bonus.

Here are Some Great Power Breakfast Choices:

- A one or two-egg omelet stuffed with plenty of veggies, some smoked turkey, and half-a-slice of light Swiss cheese (just enough for the flavor without much additional fat). Pair it with a glass of vegetable juice for even more nutrients with none of the sugar you'll find in fruit juices.

- High protein, high fiber, low sugar dry cereal such as Kashi Go Lean varieties, oatmeal squares, or wheat squares. You can mix several of them together and serve with skim milk, or unsweetened vanilla almond milk (for half the calories and double the calcium of regular skim milk). When you're on the run, put the cereal in a baggie and the milk in a travel mug. Check the labels for other cereals with high protein (5-12 grams per serving) and/or high fiber (again, usually about 5-12 grams).

- Good old-fashioned oatmeal is a fantastic and filling breakfast. The traditional canister of "Old Fashioned Oats" is highest in fiber and protein. The little packets of instant oatmeal have more sugar and less protein and fiber. Make it with water instead of milk and add cinnamon, a teaspoon of chopped nuts (and a small pinch of brown sugar if you need it). You can make your own "packets" by measuring out 1/2 cup of whole oats into baggies and adding your add-ins (raisins, nuts, spices, brown sugar) to be ready to go with water in the microwave.

- Whatever you choose for your power breakfast, I suggest packing a piece of fruit, a bag of carrots, or leftover roasted veggies for mid-morning to take you comfortably through until lunch.

Here's to a good breakfast! Power on!

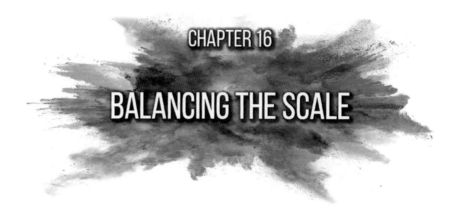

CHAPTER 16

BALANCING THE SCALE

B EING OVERWEIGHT SEEMS to be the norm in many areas and yet we can't seem to turn around the runaway train. Take another look at these shocking statistics from the Center for Disease Control (CDC) to gain an appreciation for the alarming rate at which obesity rates have increased over the past thirty years. It is truly at the point of an epidemic. We are fighting the battle of our lives—the battle against obesity.

Obesity Trends* Among U.S. Adults
BRFSS, 1990, 2000, 2010
(*BMI ≥30, or about 30 lbs. overweight for 5'4" person)

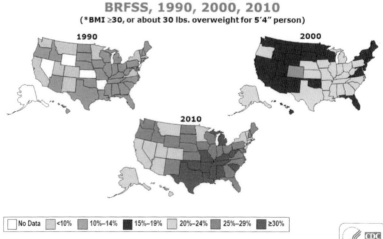

| | No Data | <10% | 10%–14% | 15%–19% | 20%–24% | 25%–29% | ≥30% |

Source: Behavioral Risk Factor Surveillance System, CDC.

We know that excess body weight is a barrier to fully realizing our potential for a strong body, a sharp brain, and endless energy. We also know that obesity is linked to an increased incidence of a host of diseases and health risks:

- Diabetes
- Heart disease
- Stroke
- High blood pressure
- Gallbladder disease
- Cancer (uterine, breast, colorectal, kidney, gall bladder and others)
- Increased surgical risk
- Osteoarthritis
- Joint pain and limited mobility
- Sleep apnea & other breathing difficulties
- Complications during pregnancy
- Menstrual irregularities
- Psychological disorders such as depression
- Stress incontinence

NEVER TOO EARLY
Balancing the Scales

Don't be blind to what you are eating. It's worth the investment to track it, even for just a few days!

NEVER TOO LATE
Balancing the Scales

If you aren't able to be very active due to mobility issues or pain, you will have a hard time expending additional calories intentionally. Those who want to lose weight will likely have to rely more on eating adjustments.

Additional statistics from the CDC link obesity or overweight with:

- 80% of Type II diabetics
- 70% of those with cardiovascular disease
- 42% of breast and colon cancer victims
- 30% of gall bladder surgeries
- 26% of obese people have high blood pressure

More CDC statistics show:

- The life expectancy of a moderately obese person could be shortened by 2-5 years.
- Obese people have a 50%—100% increased risk of death from all causes, compared with normal weight people.

- Childhood obesity is on a rise to the extent that the current generation of children is the first generation in human history who is not expected to live longer than the previous generation because of the obesity epidemic.

The good news is that as serious as it is, there are things we can do to prevent the continuing increase in obesity. Certainly, there is a genetic component that will impact our journey and expectations, but there is much within our control. The keys to losing weight are straightforward, but do require discipline, which is usually the hardest part. Being successful involves more than just "what" we need to do. Most of us would fare better if we reexamine the mental barriers that we covered earlier in this book about habit change.

We have also been conditioned to believe that it's harder to lose weight as we age. This can be true due to several reasons—hormonal changes, medications, a decrease in muscle mass that leads to a slower metabolism, and sometimes mobility problems that can reduce our opportunity to burn calories. It is lucky for us that this is not the final word. There are still many factors—in fact, the most significant factors—which we *can* impact, so we should not lose heart.

METABOLISM: EATING, BURNING, AND STORING CALORIES

At the heart of any discussion on weight and obesity is the calories in-calories out equation. It is at once simple and complex. There are many factors affecting both sides of the equation. Some you can measure, some you can't. Some you can control, some you can't.

Calories In

You may have heard your metabolism compared to a burning fire. It's a great analogy. For a fire to burn bright, you need to throw logs on the fire, correct? Our metabolism increases each time we eat. That is another reason why starving yourself or skipping meals works against you for weight loss. It slows your metabolism and causes hormonal changes that increase fat storage when you do go back to eating.

Let's be a bit more specific about the phrase "throwing a log on the fire". A huge log smothers a new fire. Kindling helps a fire catch and that is what you want for your metabolism also. Large meals smother your body with too many calories all at once. Small, frequent meals are best to help you eat a little, burn a little, then eat some more. Unfortunately, that is not typically what we see when we look around at the super-sized portions and all-you-can-eat mentalities of our society.

Calories Out

It is very tempting to equate calorie burning with exercise alone, but the reality is that our total calories burned in a day are the sum of three main components:

1. Resting metabolic rate (energy needed just to sustain life even when you are sleeping)
2. Daily activity (light to moderate moving around during the day)
3. Exercise (moderate or vigorous purposeful activity)

There is also a fourth factor in the total calories we burn in a day and that is the "thermogenic effect of food". Each time we eat, the act of digestion increases our metabolic rate. This is the reason why it's important to avoid skipping meals, especially breakfast, and to eat frequently during the day (without eating excessive calories in total). Each time we eat, we are providing stimulation for your metabolic rate.

Resting Metabolic Rate

Let's revisit some of the concepts from Chapter 11 "Just MOVE". We discussed the fact that our *resting* metabolic rate is the *largest* contributor to total caloric expenditure in a day, not exercise. Your body burns on average, approximately one calorie per minute at rest, 24 hours a day just to keep you alive. Have you heard people say they have a slow metabolism or a fast metabolism? This can be true, and someone with a "fast" metabolism might be burning a little over one calorie per minute while at rest, and someone with a slower metabolism may be burning a little less than one calorie per minute while at rest.

Individuals do vary, partially due to genetics and partially due to factors that you can control. This makes the latter one of the most important calorie-burning components to maximize, rather than assuming it's a fixed rate that can't change. We can affect it both for better and for worse.

How to increase your metabolic rate so you can burn more calories per minute:

- The simple act of eating—every time we "put a log on the fire", we stimulate our metabolism.

- Strength training exercise—The more muscle you have, the more calories you can burn all day long. Muscle is metabolically active and fat is less so, therefore, pound for pound, the more muscle you have on your body, the faster your metabolism will be.

- Aerobic exercise—When you engage in regular aerobic exercise, it causes changes within your muscle cells that burn more calories per minute all day long.

Avoid the following metabolic rate decreasing activities that cause you to burn fewer calories per minute:

- Meal skipping—Every time you skip a meal, you lose the opportunity to throw a log on your fire and your metabolic rate will stay at a lower rate.

- Dieting—Chronic calorie restriction causes hormonal changes that put your body into calorie conservation mode, making it difficult to burn calories and easier to store calories. Even when you want to lose weight, it's smart to only decrease total calories by a reasonable amount.

- Muscle loss through decreased activity over time.

Daily Activity

The next metabolic level above resting metabolism includes the calories you burn by moving around all day. This can vary quite a bit from person to person. In the "Just MOVE" section, we discussed that every time you stand up, you burn 50% more calories than when you sit, and when you walk around, you burn *twice* as many calories as when you sit.

Remember that for a few minutes or even an hour, the difference may not seem significant, but think about a comparison between someone who spends the majority of their day sitting instead of moving around. *That* is where the difference lies. Also remember that even if you exercise for one hour each day, you should ask yourself what your body is doing the "other 23 hours of the day". You can make an impact on your health by living your life in a way that seeks to *use* your body rather than seeking ways to conserve energy.

Another concept introduced in the chapter "Just MOVE" was tracking daily steps with technology like FitBits (www.FitBit.com.) I use FitBits extensively with my clients as a goal and progress checker and motivational tool. Think about all the ways your daily choices can add up!

Exercise

Although planned exercise isn't the largest contributor to overall calorie burning in a day, it is our best opportunity to burn the largest number of calories per minute for a set amount of time. During many kinds of exercise, you will burn calories at a rate of 8-12 times greater than your resting metabolic rate. That gives you good reason to add a dose of intentional exercise on most days to keep your weight in check.

Doing the Work to Lose the Pounds

Losing weight can be a long-term struggle for many people; it always seeming just out of grasp. Unfortunately, what works isn't quick or exciting. It isn't new or glamorous, either. Success in the weight loss game comes down to consistent habits over time, solid habits that you can see yourself maintaining with no end in sight. That being said, here are some tangible tips to help you on your way:

- Ditch the diets
  Any "diet" will lead to losing weight (at least temporarily) if it reduces total calories. The question is can you keep it up for the long term. The latest fad diets are almost never a good idea—they typically aren't sustainable, nor necessary for weight loss. Stick with the core weight loss principles that have stood the test of time.

- Weigh yourself daily
  One thing that can help many weight loss seekers is desensitizing themselves to the scale so it's not so scary. Daily fluctuations are normal, and it can be helpful to get in tune with your body's weight norms. Instead of burying your head in the sand, you can also course correct a lot sooner when you see things trending in the wrong direction.

- Use a food log and an activity tracker together.
  We've already reviewed the merits of websites like MyFitnessPal and technology like the FitBit. Real magic can occur when you use them together. This is the closest you'll get to reconciling your calories in with your calories out. Following a set of realistic goals consistently will increase your likelihood of long-term success.

Many of us have so much to gain from losing!

STEP FIVE:

BEYOND EATING
AND EXERCISE

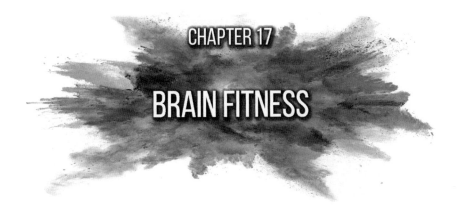

CHAPTER 17

BRAIN FITNESS

BRAIN HEALTH AND mental sharpness are not just a concern for older adults. As with physical fitness, it is never too early or too late to prioritize brain fitness. Starting early is important for improving mental performance markers such as intellectual ability, mental clarity, processing speed, both short-term and long-term memory, and reducing the risk of diseases such as Alzheimer's and other forms of dementia.

Even later in life, you haven't missed your chance to improve brain function. The term neuroplasticity is the capacity of the brain to reorganize itself and create new neural pathways. The brain is an amazing organ which indeed retains neuroplasticity throughout life—it grows and responds to stimuli at any age, just as your muscles adapt to physical training. It used to be commonly thought that brain functions were destined to steadily decline with age, but that does not have to be the case. Change, renewal, and improvement are possible after brain injury, disease, or advanced age.

Many people do experience changes in brain function as they age. Almost 40% of people over the age of 65 experience some memory loss. Mild cognitive changes, however, are different than Alzheimer's and other forms of dementia, which are diseases. Some estimates predict that the number of Americans over the age of 65 with Alzheimer's disease could more than triple from 5 million to 16 million by the year 2050! As with physical health, the increased prevalence of impairments in brain health are largely due to *lifestyle* factors—the *same ones* that harm our physical health; things like diet, exercise, sleep, stress, and much more.

Strategies to Sharpen Your Brain

The "use it or lose it" principle applies to the mind as well as the body and there are many things we can do to improve our brain function throughout our lives.

1. Physical Exercise

The number one way to make your brain sharper is physical exercise! This is an important point to take to heart because it's a common misconception that the best way to improve brain function is through brain exercises. By now, you should not be surprised that physical exercise tops the list. Our Magic Pill strikes again!

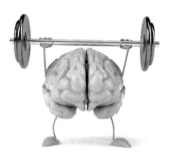

Exercise increases blood flow to the brain and reduces your risk of dementia by 30-40%. What a huge incentive alone to exercise! Exercise also reduces your risk of depression and high cholesterol which are both also linked to dementia. Strength training has been shown to improve memory along with a multitude of other benefits.

Composite of 20 student brains taking the same test

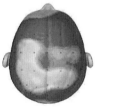
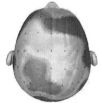

After sitting quietly   After 20 minute walk

Research/Scan compliments of Dr. Chuck Hillman University of Illinois

2. Physical Exercise and Brain Exercise at the Same Time

There are some studies that show that asking the brain to think *while* performing physical exercise provides a double stimulus for powerful brain function improvement. Examples of this would be a dance class where you need to remember the steps while you are moving as opposed to walking or riding a stationary bike that does not require any thinking.

3. Brain Exercises

There is definitely a place for brain exercises such as crossword puzzles, Sudoku, online memory games and specific brain fitness exercises. Practice challenging your brain on a regular basis!

4. Nutrition

The Superfoods are just as powerful for improving our brain health as they are for improving our physical health and energy. Here's the list again. Eat more of these:

SUPERFOODS		
Tomatoes	Spinach	Yogurt
Broccoli	Whole Grains	Salmon
Sweet Potatoes	Edamame	Quinoa
Avocado	Winter Squashes	Barley
Pumpkin	Nuts and Seeds	Farro
Beans	Leafy greens	Berries
Lentils	Flax Seed	

In addition, it's important to eat a high fiber, low fat, and low cholesterol diet for a healthy brain, as high cholesterol is a risk factor for dementia.

5. Sleep

During sleep, the flow of cerebrospinal fluid in the brain increases dramatically, washing away harmful toxins, namely a waste protein called beta-amyloid, that creates plaques in the brain linked to Alzheimer's. Therefore, getting enough sleep can reduce the risk of Alzheimer's. Sleep is vital for tissue repair, rejuvenation, and memory retention!

6. Challenging Your Brain and Learning Something New
Whether it's a new language, a musical instrument, or a class on art or history, embracing the challenge (and frustration) of learning something new has a remarkable benefit to the brain. It's easy to think classes are in the past once you have surpassed school-age, but there are many exciting models and opportunities for adult education. Give some thought to something you've always wanted to learn about and jump in!

7. Continually Change Your Routine
The brain's pathways can resemble a well-worn path through a grassy field when you do the same things the same way all the time. Changing your daily routine by driving a different route to work or brushing your teeth with your non-dominant hand will force your brain to create new nerve connections and new pathways. New nerve pathways are brain growth!

NEVER TOO EARLY Brain Fitness

Brain fitness is not only for older adults. We should start early with these important habits, just as with our physical fitness.

NEVER TOO LATE Brain Fitness

Brain fitness is a primary concern of many older adults. Take heed of this chapter as an important one!

8. Stress Reduction
When we are under stress, the body secretes excess amounts of cortisol and other stress hormones. Cortisol has been shown to damage the hippocampus, which is the memory center of the brain. This is especially significant for older adults since the size of the hippocampus reduces in older age by as much as 20%. It's easy to think stress is just part of life or to tell yourself you'll relax after whatever stressful event is going on in your life is over. The trouble is that once one situation resolves, there's usually something else on its heels. The key is to learn strategies

for managing stress day to day and especially during the storms of life. I'll cover that in an upcoming section of this book.

9. Social Connections
Relationships and social stimulation are good for the brain. Challenge yourself to branch out socially and take some risks. The larger and more complex our social networks, the larger the amygdala becomes (which plays a major role in behavior and motivation). Also, when we hug someone or experience other meaningful human touch, it releases the hormone oxytocin, which suppresses the release of cortisol (the hormone that damages the brain). Hug therapy for brain fitness sounds amazing!

10. Purpose
What's your reason for getting up in the morning? What excites you? Oftentimes, we hear about people who have cognitive decline after retiring because they lose their purpose and stimulation of their brain and social lives. Of course, it doesn't have to be this way. Many people are using their retirement years for new adventures. Regardless of your age, why not reflect on how your daily life matches up with a greater sense of purpose and if there's a gap, give some thought to what would excite you!

11. Variety, Surprise, and Zeal
When the body is presented with an overload in an exercise setting, it adapts and grows to meet the challenge placed upon it. The brain is the same. Look for ways to inject your daily life with variety, surprise, and zeal for new things to keep your brain guessing.

12. Healthy Hearing
Hearing is a very important part of the five senses. When you experience hearing loss, the brain is robbed of important stimulation on an ongoing basis, resulting in less opportunity for growth. The link between hearing loss and dementia is

significant. With each 10-decibel loss of hearing, dementia risk increases by 20%. Mild hearing loss doubles the risk of dementia. Moderate hearing loss triples the risk, and severe hearing loss increases the risk of dementia five times!

The relationship between healthy hearing and brain loss is so significant; let's examine it further.

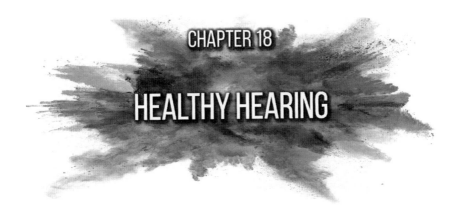

CHAPTER 18

HEALTHY HEARING

Healthy hearing is one of the most important things we need to protect for a sharp brain because hearing loss leads to a reduction in sensory input to our brain, which in turn leads to reduced cognitive functioning. It also follows along with our theme of never too early and never too late. Even young people can have problems with their hearing due to headphones, concerts, and other habits. Early detection and intervention are crucial in protecting and preserving your ability to hear.

I'm not an audiologist and until a few years ago, healthy hearing was not at all on my radar for wellness. That all changed when I met Eve at a retirement community. Eve suffered from significant hearing loss. She was an advocate for awareness and intervention for hearing loss and I admired her great zeal and determination. She exposed me to data that was so shocking and compelling that she turned me into an advocate as well. After getting to know Eve, I began including healthy hearing in all my wellness-related educational efforts because of its importance and integral fit, and because of what seems to be a gaping hole in awareness and attention. The scope of the problem and the profound effects of hearing loss are not adequately appreciated. Consider the following statistics:

- 50% of 65-year-olds have hearing loss.

- 80% of 85-year-olds have hearing loss.

- People with hearing loss are not aware of what they don't hear and thus, their comprehension of the interactions around them is deficient.

- Most people wait an average of seven years of difficulty hearing before seeking treatment.

- Even then, only 20-25% ever seek treatment with hearing aids. This may be because hearing aids are often not covered by medical insurance, which is mind-boggling.

- During the time that hearing loss is being ignored, cognitive function declines. Age-related hearing loss is generally progressive, and individuals may be unaware of the severity of the progression. Early detection and treatment can help retain cognitive function.

- Many people with hearing loss become so exhausted and frustrated in social settings trying to communicate that they start tuning out or choosing to stay home more often. This leads to social isolation, which can then lead to loneliness and depression, all of which have a negative impact on our physical health, brain health, energy level, and overall quality of life.

- The stress and depression from hearing loss can cause an increase in inflammation throughout the body, which can increase our risk for other diseases like cancer and heart disease.

- Hearing loss increases your risk of dementia:
  - Each 10-decibel loss = 20% increase in risk
  - Mild hearing loss = double the risk
  - Moderate hearing loss = triple the risk
  - Severe hearing loss = five times the risk

- Many people are in denial about their hearing loss because there is a stigma about hearing loss and hearing aids as a stereotype of unattractive aging.

- Help is available, including simple tips, strategies, and technologies that can significantly improve hearing and quality of life. Those with hearing loss shouldn't settle for not hearing and/or staying at home.

- Be prepared that improvements require an investment of time and money.
  - See an audiologist to get tested.
  - If you are prescribed hearing aids, wear them! (Many people don't.)
  - Unlike eyeglasses, hearing aids need ongoing adjustments and maintenance so be prepared to address issues. It's worth it! If your hearing aids are uncomfortable or problematic, make an appointment with your audiologist.

- Look into other technologies and devices that exist to supplement hearing. There are more and newer products every year.

- Take advantage of situational strategies that will improve your quality of life if you have hearing loss and/or wear hearing aids. If your family member has hearing loss, there is much you can do to facilitate better hearing in social situations:

  NEVER TOO EARLY
  Healthy Hearing
  If you've been exposed to loud sounds or excessive headphone usage, have your hearing checked.

  NEVER TOO LATE
  Healthy Hearing
  This is a super important chapter for older adults! Read it carefully!

  - Don't shout or whisper. Use a strong, clear voice.
  - Look directly at the person you are speaking to, so they can watch your lips move.
  - When dining, choose tables of four or less and only one person should speak at a time. Large parties and people talking on top of one another is difficult to manage for those with hearing loss.

- ○ Request microphone use when it's available.
- ○ For churches, auditoriums, and other large venues, check to see if they have a "hearing loop" that your hearing aid can tap into.
- ○ Move conversations to a quieter place that limits background noise.

Here is a quote from "Peter", another advocate for hearing loss who I've had the pleasure of knowing. I think of him often and admire his dedication:

> "Every year it becomes a little easier and more attractive to stop fighting (participating) and just drop out of the various battles. Fortunately, we are beginning to learn that one must stay engaged despite all the increasingly depressing frustrations. The alternative is oblivion."

Do whatever you can to preserve your healthy hearing.

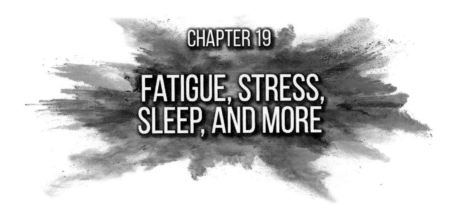

CHAPTER 19

FATIGUE, STRESS, SLEEP, AND MORE

FATIGUE IS A universal feeling we can all relate to but perhaps there is a point of view that is different and gives us new insights on how to overcome it. The temptation is to seek a shortcut or supplement that will give us more energy—a vitamin, or energy drink, or caffeine. Rather than looking for an outside source, consider that our own bodies have the power within already. Entertain the notion that how we feel may be due to a combination of many, small, separately less significant factors that we take for granted. Separately, they are each just one more thing we know we should do, but together, they spell vibrancy or fatigue.

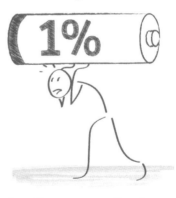

There are four factors that make a significant contribution to fatigue. A few are obvious; a few are not. Strive to get the basics right by addressing these four culprits, rather than ignoring them and looking for an outside source of energy on the shelves of a supplement store.

1. SLEEP DEPRIVATION

It's common practice to steal nighttime hours for daytime activities and to underestimate the value of sleep. Of course, we are starting with the obvious in stating that lack of sleep causes fatigue, but there are some eye-opening (no pun intended!) statistics that reveal just how dangerous our lack of sleep can be. Getting enough sleep is as important to a strong body, sharp brain, and endless energy as exercise and eating well. According to the National Sleep Foundation:

- One-third of the population is sleeping less than 6 hours per night which causes you to be 50% more likely to be overweight.

- Roughly 40 million Americans suffer from sleep disorders.

- 27% of adults have dozed off at the wheel.

- Sleep deprivation accelerates the aging process.

- Lack of sleep weakens your immune system.

- Lack of sleep hinders memory consolidation and the removal of plaques in the brain.

Yikes! Anyone else feel alarmed and committed to getting more zzzs? What are some tips for getting better sleep?

NEVER TOO EARLY
Fatigue, Stress, and Sleep

You are not invincible. Even if you don't necessarily feel bad or think you can get by until life eases up, think again. Often, negative things are happening inside our bodies that we can't see. Take care of yourself!

NEVER TOO LATE
Fatigue, Stress, and Sleep

These are such important issues as we age. The consequences may feel magnified and be a good incentive to take these areas seriously.

- Keep regular bed/wake times if possible.

- Protect your sleep time. Avoid working in your bedroom.

- If you drink caffeine, have a caffeine cut-off time several hours prior to bedtime.

- Gauge your sensitivity to screen time in the evenings and avoid it in bed.

2. STRESS

Stress takes quite a toll on the body, both physically and psychologically. Anyone who's had the experience of a significant stressor knows that it utterly drains you. (Think planning a wedding, surviving a family rift, or dealing with the loss of a loved one.) Yet, we often don't recognize that daily, run-of-the-mill stress also has an impact. Of course, not all stress is bad. When stress is part of an acute situation and is at a manageable level, it drives us to get things done. When stress is chronic and/or the level is unmanageable, it leads to burnout and disease.

How can stress impair your health and your energy?

- Stress causes your liver to increase cholesterol production and increases your blood pressure, which increases your risk of heart disease.

- Stress can also lead you to eat less healthfully, which can also increase weight and cholesterol.

- Stress hormones such as cortisol are released at a higher rate, causing weight gain, high blood pressure, and an increased risk of diabetes.

- These stress hormones also harm your brain and weaken the immune system, increasing your risk of getting sick.

Taking action to manage stress in your daily life is an important step to boosting your energy quotient. What are some tips for managing stress?

- Take stock and make a personal "stress-less" strategy. Are you overcommitted? Look at what you have on your plate and what you might want to adjust or remove if it no longer fits with your priorities. Another option is to re-examine your priorities based on the impact that stress is having on your health and quality of life.

- Give yourself an attitude adjustment called "seeing your choices": If the stressor is something you can control, what action can you take? Feeling in control helps a lot.

If it's something you can't control, what thought pattern can you change? Remember, our thoughts cause our feelings. Have you heard the saying, "What you focus on grows"? Whether it's the positive view or the negative view, you are making it "grow" when you think about it.

- Buffer yourself to stay strong against daily stressors with healthy eating, exercise, making time for relaxation, and getting enough sleep.

- Cultivate teamwork and positive communication with your relationships. Many stressful situations are relationship issues.

- Pick a few "stress busters" as your go-to tools for regular usage and also for those particularly stressful situations:
    o Deep breathing (It really works!)
    o Exercise (of COURSE!)
    o Call a friend
    o Massage, tai chi, visualization, progressive relaxation, prayer, or meditation
    o Community Service (focusing on others take your worry off yourself)

Are you a resilient person?

Resilience is a concept worth thinking about. There is no magic wand to remove stress. We need to break our chronic stress patterns to keep stress from wreaking havoc with our health. Stress-resistant people view life differently than stress-prone people. Qualities to cultivate include being flexible, optimistic, action-oriented, a moderate risk-taker, open with others, self-confident, connected to others, and accepting of support. That's quite a list to attack all at once, especially when you feel overwhelmed. Try picking one quality at a time to focus on. You can also think about these four Cs as a way to reframe life experiences to build resilience: Challenges, Commitment, Control, and Courage!

3. DEHYDRATION

Does it surprise you that dehydration is a source of fatigue? Fluids play a crucial role in almost all bodily functions, yet many of us go hours without drinking anything when we're busy. The simple fact is that water is necessary to keep those billions of cells plumped up, humming along, and your energy levels consistent. While all non-caffeinated beverages and foods that have a high water content can count towards your fluid intake, water is the best source of hydration—free of calories, sugar, and caffeine. If you are serious about increasing your energy level, and improving your skin, muscles, brain function, and more, you will make a plan to stay hydrated.

What patterns can you set up to help you increase your water consumption? Try some of the below:

- Drink a full glass of water upon rising in the morning.
- Drink water frequently before, during, and after exercise.
- Drink water with every meal.
- Fill a large water bottle in the morning to keep with you throughout the day with a goal of finishing it before dinner.
- Drink another full glass of water every evening at some point. (It doesn't have to be too close to bedtime if you are concerned with getting up in the middle of the night to use the bathroom.)

4. INACTIVITY

Nature's own remedy for fatigue is exercise and it doesn't cost a cent. Exercise equals energy, period. There is nothing quite like moving your muscles to get oxygen into your lungs and coursing through your body. Increased oxygen usage is vibrancy and cell renewal at its best. With exercise, you invigorate your muscles and your brain. Feel-good hormones abound. They don't call it "runner's high" for nothing!

You might be saying "But I don't have the energy to exercise!" It's a "chicken and the egg" questions, isn't it? You know that exercise will *give* you energy, but you don't have the energy to exercise. Try these tips:

- Start small. If you don't feel like exercising, tell yourself you'll do just five minutes. Next thing you know, you may decide that since you're already doing it, you might as well go a bit longer.

- Give more consideration to the time of day that you try to exercise and match that to your personality and natural body rhythms. Many people find that exercising first thing in the morning gives them the best chance at being consistent. Others know themselves and are not early birds. They know that their body is at its best in the late afternoon. You could also try varying the time of day you exercise until you find what works best.

- Get out there and just walk. Exercise doesn't get any simpler than lacing up and hitting a brisk pace for even just ten or fifteen minutes. You'll be amazed at how great you feel.

- Link a simple exercise to another activity that is already part of your daily routine. No one reminds you to brush your teeth. You could do push-ups on the bathroom vanity every morning right after brushing your teeth. Before long, it will be second nature rather than one more thing to remember.

Give some new habits a try. You've got nothing to lose, and plenty of energy to gain! We all want more energy. Commit to going back to the basics. Even more to the point, trust your body. You don't need any special pills or potions. It's kind of like the "Everything I Ever Needed to Know I Learned in Kindergarten" message. Too often, we underestimate the value of the basics or just neglect them and hope we can fix it with something we can buy and ingest. Manage stress, drink plenty of water, get some exercise, and get some sleep. It's nothing your mother hasn't already told you and it works!

AND MORE

As we get to the end of step five, there are a few other self-care practices that shouldn't be ignored in our quest for a strong body, sharp brain, and endless energy.

Smoking

Smoking, or rather *not* smoking is a key element for achieving all three of our goals. The health risks of smoking are of course no secret. If you are currently a smoker, remember that smoking *less* is valuable, even if you don't feel able to quit altogether right now. If you feel ready to tackle this area of your life, talk to your doctor for assistance. There are medications and programs that can be helpful. Most smokers are not successful quitting on their first attempt, so if you would like to be smoke-free, don't give up!

Self-Care

While it is beyond the scope of this book, please be sure to see your doctor on a regular basis for screenings that are appropriate for you (such as cholesterol, blood pressure, mammograms, prostate, and more). Unfortunately, many individuals don't have a primary care physician. Did you know that having a personal relationship with a primary care physician is one of the best ways to protect your health? When you see your physician regularly for check-ups, you'll have a partner in your health journey who will make sure you receive screenings and care at the right intervals as you progress through the stages of life.

Make sure your wellness is well-rounded!

STEP SIX:

ACROSS THE AGES—WITH EACH OTHER

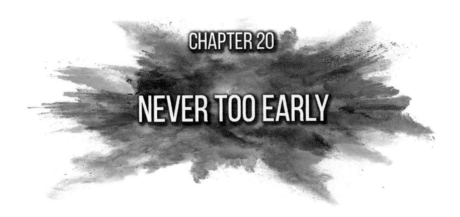

CHAPTER 20

NEVER TOO EARLY

CHILDHOOD

IT IS TRULY never too early to prioritize habits that lead to a strong body, sharp brain, and endless energy. When we have babies, toddlers, and preschoolers, the parental instinct is at its strongest for ensuring that our children get enough sleep, eat healthy foods, and move their bodies in developmentally appropriate ways.

Once a child reaches school-age (but sometimes younger), the ease and allure of fast food and processed snack foods can become an issue. Screen time, in its expanding forms, is often at such an excessive level that it qualifies as an addiction. What's the answer? Parents can do their children a huge favor by implementing strategies early to make healthier foods more available and less healthy foods less available.

The standard excuses of being too busy to cook at home or assuming "that's all they'll eat" about hot dogs and mac-and-cheese needs to be challenged if we are going to stand a chance in reversing the shocking increase in childhood obesity. Extreme health efforts won't work with kids, however, and often have the reverse effect. Kids who are kept on very strict diets at home are often the first to go overboard in settings without parental supervision. We all know what moderation looks like and we'll do our children a world of good by setting (and sticking to) screen time limits, facilitating opportunities for physical activity, especially as a family, and making healthy food and healthy habits part of our family's way of life.

> Matt (17) loves soccer more than anything. He will wake up in the early morning if there's a soccer game being played in England that he needs to watch in real-time. His own workout habits are centered around improving his soccer performance. Running, check. If you don't have cardiovascular endurance, you can't be the first one to the ball. Weight training, check. He needs power in his legs and core. He's also fond of "juggling" the ball around the house, practicing his coordination and ball control skills. I'm glad he is building a good base for the next phase of his life!

> Dylan (16) is always up for trying something new and he's always a trooper. As a freshman in high school, he tried cross country in the fall, since his older brothers loved it. It was great to prepare him for the winter sports season when he wanted to try wrestling for the first time. His assessment? Not "fun" at all, but it was challenging and confidence-building, and showed him what his body is capable of. Spring brought a third new sport to try—rugby! Now THIS, he said was pure fun; a bunch of guys running and tackling with very few rules. He's building an adventurous spirit and great habits for his future!

COLLEGE STUDENTS AND YOUNG ADULTS

Going off to college is an important transition time for an older teen. What type of routines are they going to create for themselves once their time is their own to schedule? Will they fall prey to the "freshman 15" pound weight gain due to an all-you-can-eat dining hall setting and delivery pizza like I did?

We can help our young adults by setting healthy examples starting years earlier. Did we only cart them around to their sports activities or did we stay active ourselves? We can also stay in close touch to help strategize and lend a supportive ear.

We all create our unique routines through trial and error, but the examples we see and the encouragement we receive can make a big impact on the priorities we set. One positive aspect of college dining halls is that in their goal of having something for everyone, there are almost always plentiful healthy choices for those who desire them. College campuses also brim with opportunities for recreational sports, exercise, and willing companions for these activities.

The transition from college-age student or young adult living at home to working and becoming a self-supporting adult can be a challenging one, and it's probably one of the most important transitions for instilling life-long habits.

Many young people find that "adulting" is so time-consuming that the more active recreational activities from their college or living-at-home days are no longer as easy to fit in. They might also categorize those activities as part of what "kids" do, like play on an organized sports team or attend a P.E. class. They might fall into a habit of eating out or going to happy hour too often and suddenly find themselves in a situation where their waistline is showing a change.

It can be difficult to manage your bills, care for a pet, buy groceries, keep your home clean, and so much more when you have been used to someone else shouldering so many of these boring, time-consuming errands and tasks. The answers again are routine and support during this transitional phase. Grocery shopping and meal-planning advice and setting an exercise routine that is realistic given their new schedule can be a huge help. Young adults can benefit from their parents or other trusted adults serving as a sounding board and example of healthy habits that can serve them well for many years to come.

Another common scenario of young adulthood is the feeling of being invincible. It's true that youth is very forgiving of bad habits and it's a bit easier to look good and feel fine even when your habits aren't great. Even so, start now if you haven't already. Years have a way of flying by and the habits that you set now can build a foundation for when life becomes even more demanding.

> Jenna (23) has been out of college for a few years and has taken a unique (and enviable!) path by moving to Paris. With a career in the hospitality industry, she spends a lot of time on her feet and does not have traditional 9-5 hours. She has learned to adapt and fit in exercise when she can. She's a fan of keeping things simple, with brisk walking and simple weight training. She's also a healthy eater (despite her occasional sweet tooth that she inherited from her mother). She is methodical and goal-oriented, so she gets done what is needed and that will take her far.

> Tyler (23), graduated from Virginia Military Institute and commissioned into the Army. He has always been drawn to the more rigorous physical challenges that the military is known for (to which I say, better him than me!) Running cross country in high school gave him a great foundation and adding weight training through college has made him a formidable force, which is exactly what is needed for him to

confidently assume his responsibilities. The discipline and fitness-minded culture of the military will serve him well for his health through the years!

Jeff (21) inspires me with his fitness drive. He has loved running since the 3rd grade when he was one of the fastest kids in his class in the one-mile run. He has never been afraid to push himself. On the soccer field, he would sprint from play to play, red-faced but never out of energy. When he made the transition to cross country in high school, I never saw anyone work harder or gain more healthy habits such as eating healthy foods when no one else was and drinking water all day. Cross country success doesn't come only from practices during the season, but your pre-season discipline and early morning runs. When he arrived at Purdue on a NROTC scholarship, his high level of conditioning from cross country was above most of his peers. This put him in the position of a fitness mentor, encouraging the others and leading workouts. One fantastic practice he told me about is his participation in the H.E.R.O. club with many of his ROTC friends. They select a fallen soldier, create a challenging workout that honors him, and push themselves to complete it while thinking about him. Afterward, they send a letter and photos to the soldier's loved ones letting them know what they did. What a wonderful thing to do to bring incredible meaning and motivation to a workout and keep the memory alive for someone who made the ultimate sacrifice for our country.

WORKING ADULTS

Oftentimes, our twenties fly by while we have all the time in the world, the thirties become a blur while we raise a young family, and the forties can be the busiest time with our careers and possibly raising teenagers. Of course, life patterns vary greatly, but when I question people about the passage of time, almost everyone says "I can't believe I'm already *this* old"—*whatever* age that is. The passage of time will only feel more rapid as we get older (or so I hear) and trouble can sneak up as the years go by.

I once had a client in her forties tell me, "It's not hard to look good when you are younger, but as I've aged, I notice it becoming more difficult. I look around at women a bit older than me and I can tell who's been putting in the work and who hasn't. This same phenomenon happens at high school reunions (or graduation year Facebook pages) since they are petri dishes of people who are exactly the same chronological age but who have aged differently. Haven't we all noticed someone who we thought has or has not "aged well"?

I find it odd how some people in their forties or fifties start complaining about being old. Those decades are *not* "old". Aches and pains in those decades are not a given. Remember the philosophy *"once you think something is inevitable, you stop trying to prevent it"*. The gradual slip and slide of health and vitality through middle adulthood is not the only scenario, as we've been discussing since page one. Taking a serious approach to the principles of a strong body, sharp brain, and endless energy can be truly life changing.

One important caution for working-age adults is to be careful of falling into a situation of "can't see the forest for the trees". When we keep our focus on small, everyday to-do items, it's easy to miss the big picture. The core "never too early" philosophy and strategies are targeted at younger or middle-aged adults. Start now, regardless of your age, in order to improve your health, appearance, and quality of life now and for the future decades of your life.

My husband Matt is a true outdoorsman. His idea of a great time on the weekends is to head up to his hunting trailer in rural PA and "clear land". I tease him that he's going up there to pick up sticks, but having an active hobby is fantastic as we age. He could spend all day losing track of time while chopping down trees and splitting wood. His other trick is wearing what he calls his "Ninja clothes" under his work clothes during the week so that if it's a nice day, he can be ready to fit in a run at lunchtime. File that away as "whatever works"!

BUSY PARENTS

Whether busy parents are working outside of the home or not, they are often the most squeezed for time and suffer the most from physical and mental fatigue. Raising children can be one of the most rewarding things you ever do, while being very depleting at the same time if you aren't careful.

I wrote and published *The Busy Mom's Ultimate Fitness Guide* in 2006 while I was a young mother. At the time, my three children were 11, 9, and 5 and I could certainly relate to the challenges of living a healthy life while raising children.

One of the benefits of figuring out a healthy living routine when you have children is setting an example for them of healthy habits *and* an example of the world not totally revolving around them. One risk that some parents fall into is being so child-focused that they do not leave any time for themselves. This can inadvertently send the wrong message to children that their parents' entire role is to cater to their children's needs. Isn't it much better for children to see the example of parents caring for their children *and* themselves? Certainly, it's not easy, but as we've discussed, when it's a priority and you don't have an all-or-none attitude, you can figure out a plan that makes sense and is valuable.

People are often curious about my own exercise habits since it's what I talk about for a living. I love to exercise first thing in the morning before anything else can interfere. I find it to be the best way to start the day! It's not easy to juggle it with driving the kids to school, but it's better than leaving it to happen or not happen later in the day. I have all the equipment I need in my basement exercise room and that saves me a lot of time. I'm pretty no-nonsense about my workouts. I usually do something cardiovascular 6-7 days per week but I'm careful not to overstress my joints. I mix up running, brisk walking, using an elliptical, and heading up to the local pool for deep water running. I typically do my strength training three days per week. My favorite workouts are running with my husband, taking a long brisk walk with my neighbor to catch up, or watching a favorite show I've taped and saved to watch while I'm on the elliptical. Recently, I've added an extra focus on stretching which helps my muscles and joints feel so much more comfortable during the day. I am certain that exercise elevates my mood!

Don't let the years go by in a blur without prioritizing your strong body, sharp brain, and endless energy!

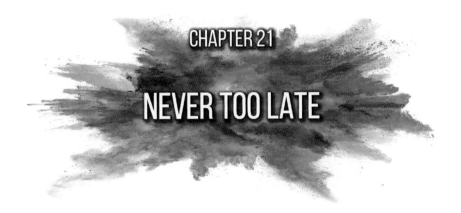

CHAPTER 21

NEVER TOO LATE

A FTER SPENDING MANY years in the company of thousands of older adults, my resolve about the possibilities of change and improving our quality of life at any age is stronger than ever. I have seen countless examples across a wide continuum of aging scenarios.

THE MAGIC PILL AS WE AGE

Yes, it's true that aging can bring physiological and cognitive changes that might be unwelcome, but remember that exercise (our Magic Pill) and other lifestyle habits can help tremendously. Our maximal oxygen capacity decreases as we age; exercise increases it. Lung capacity may reduce with age. The lungs and connective tissue become less elastic and the respiratory muscles become shortened and weakened. Exercise makes breathing easier as it stretches and strengthens these muscles and increases lung capacity. Our bones and muscles weaken as we age; exercise increases both.

Exercise also strengthens our tendons and ligaments which keep our joints supple, preserving physical independence and mobility. Exercise can help manage back pain, arthritis, and other musculoskeletal conditions, increase our resting metabolic rate, reduce our risk of diabetes and cancer, reduce stress, depression, and anxiety, improve posture, flexibility, and strengthen our immune system. This is, of course, not a definitive list and I've already said this in earlier chapters, however, the purpose of repeating these specific examples here is that they are *all* problems associated with aging. It's time for yet another reminder that our *lifestyle* choices, and specifically *exercise*, can ease or counteract each of them. Let that sink in. It does bear repeating that as we age, we simply *cannot* afford not to be exercising! *It is not too late, and you will see results.*

STAGES OF OLDER ADULTHOOD

When we think of the "never too late" population and time of life, it can be helpful to discuss two separate periods of older adulthood: those in their sixties and early seventies (current baby boomers) and those in their later seventies and older.

When we are in our sixties and early seventies, it's time to truly embrace the philosophy that what you are doing now will help you live longer and improve the quality of your life into the older years of eighties and even 90s. Negative thinking about the likelihood of living to see your 90s has no place in your plan. Healthy habits now can help give you *decades* more of life to enjoy. What a gift you can give yourself and your family members!

When we are in our late seventies, eighties and 90s, many people have some type of health concerns that they need to manage, however, there is excitement in the still present ability to positively impact your longevity and quality of life by your habits. Many people in this age range truly cherish every day and bring positivity to all they do. They can be a positive influence and an inspiration to others by the way they live their lives. This can be especially helpful in circles where older adults spend a lot of time complaining about their health problems and propagating negativity. Be the one who spreads the hope and good vibes!

NUTRITION FOR OLDER ADULTS

This book does not address specific nutritional needs of older adults because in taking a broad-brush approach, younger and older adults can benefit from the same healthy eating style. The difference is that for older adults, it can matter more, meaning when you don't follow healthy eating recommendations, you are more likely to have problems. When you are younger, it's still a good idea, but if you don't, the consequences might not catch up with you right away.

If you discuss specific nutritional needs with your physician or a registered dietitian, you can easily incorporate them into a regular routine. Likewise, addressing the specific strategies for common medical conditions is beyond the scope of this book, but lucky for us, credible information is not difficult to find, and the healthy living and exercise recommendations outlined here are generally helpful for almost all of them.

WHERE YOU LIVE MATTERS

Where do you call home? Where you live matters for your longevity and quality of life. I made up a little saying to encompass the keys you need to consider for quality of life as we age.

Cathy's Four Keys to a Healthy Living Location:
- Body
- Brain
- People
- Purpose

Does where you live provide convenient access to:

- BODY: Take care of your body? This would include healthy food (prepared for you if you are no longer able or interested in cooking for yourself), exercise opportunities, and medical care or caregiver assistance with daily living should you need it.

- BRAIN: Take care of your brain? This would include educational opportunities like classes, seminars, discussion groups, and exciting challenges should you want to partake.

- PEOPLE: Social Opportunities? Meaningful social connection is one of the important factors for longevity, quality of life, and brain health. Are you sitting alone in the same home in which you raised your children without a social network or things to do? Do you have access to clubs, luncheon groups, group outings, and more?

- PURPOSE: Meaningful pursuits? Having a purpose when you get up in the morning is also strongly linked to longevity and brain health. Do you have committees you can join if you so wish, access to the arts, a hobby, politics or volunteering if that is what energizes you?

Many older adults enjoy a setting for all of the above by moving to a 55+/senior living community. You will often find:

- More plentiful and convenient fitness opportunities and health care resources.

- More educational opportunities to stimulate your brain.

- More plentiful and structured opportunities to have purposeful pursuits—whether it be a volunteer program, woodworking studio, poetry club, resident governance committee, and much more.

- Social opportunities similar to living in a college dorm. Dinner parties and plenty of peers are the norm.

- You'll also find relief from many of the common chores of homeownership that you may be eager to give up or that you are unable to continue managing, such as lawn care, home maintenance, and cooking. Once these tasks are no longer on your plate, many people feel a new sense of freedom to travel or take up new interests.

If that doesn't sound appealing or like a good fit for you, there are other ways to accomplish the same goals. There are many community efforts and neighborhood initiatives that you could join. Once you start looking into the possibilities, you might be surprised about what is available. The important thing is to know what you value in your living arrangement as you age and to plan in advance as much as possible. Making a move at a time of crisis, such as when a spouse dies or if you are faced with a new urgent medical situation is much more stressful. In addition, we don't usually make the best decisions or have plentiful choices when we are rushed.

What About Home Care?

Some older adults find that they need assistance with daily living tasks such as taking medications, dressing, or bathing but do not want to move out of their current home. Home Care agencies can provide both medical and non-medical services in your own home. One of the most rewarding aspects of hiring a home caregiver is the relationship that can develop between the caregiver, the client, and family members. Quite often, the caregiver becomes like another family member. Consider this as opportunity to work on wellness together between the caregiver and the client!

I've heard it said that your income will be the average of the ten people you interact with the most. I think the same is true for attitude. If you surround yourself with people who are constantly complaining about the aches and pains of aging, it infiltrates you. If you choose to surround yourself with positive people who are savoring their later years and looking for the positive, then that is what will rub off on you. You could also decide to be the one that starts a positive domino effect on those around you! We are all aging. The alternative, of course, is less desirable, so embrace it and make the best of it!

> Joe and Nancy are the parents of some childhood friends. I recently bumped into Joe at a nearby 55+ community where they have been living and he looked great. I recognized his voice before I even saw him and when I turned around, there was that same Boston accent and warm smile that I remembered from years ago. He shared with me that at the age of 86, thanks to his regular fitness routine, he is able to continue playing regular golf with his buddies and he can still beat his age every now and then! I separately bumped into Nancy at the local indoor pool. She is using aquatic exercise at the recommendation of her physical therapist and she is also staying in shape and looking great!
>
> Edith is 93 and quite a mover and shaker at the retirement community where she lives. She is involved in more committees and initiatives than I can count, but what stuck out for me the first time I met her was her main reason for keeping up with her fitness routine. As a lifelong Penn State season ticket holder, she wanted to make sure she would be able to climb the bleachers with her children and grandchildren every year. So far, so good!
>
> Barbara is a retired technical manager consultant who has been successfully managing her Multiple Sclerosis (MS) diagnosis for over 30 years. I have watched her courageously plow forward with a regular exercise routine for the past eight years that I've known her. Does she love it? Not exactly, but she always has a sly smile and a joke for the fitness center team members who have supported

her. Her doctor told her that he is convinced that if she had not been exercising all these years, surely, her MS would have had her in a wheelchair by now, but on she walks. She's an inspiration!

Mary M. was one of my very first personal training clients many years ago who has since passed away. She was an older relative who had Parkinson's disease and very limited mobility. I would stop by her apartment on my way home from classes at the University of Maryland. Using soup cans and elastic tubing, we worked on the range of motion of her joints and her strength. I have great memories of her shy smile and little chuckle. I think she was humoring me in my budding career, but I know that she benefited from the exercise.

Mary H. was an avid swimmer for many years in her sixties, seventies, and eighties. When her health began to falter in her late eighties, she moved to an assisted living facility, but she didn't give up on her exercise regime. She transitioned to doing timed walks up and down her hallways with her walker and doing strength training with a personal trainer twice a week, under the supervision of a physical therapist who factors in her complicated medical history.

Sally, at 78, has been courageously fighting cancer for several years and has been determined to keep her slight frame as strong as possible through weight training exercise, supervised by a personal trainer and a physical therapist. Taking into account her energy level and chemotherapy schedule, she has good days and bad days to manage, but she never gives up!

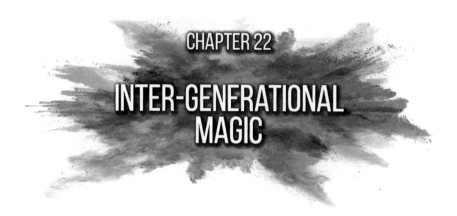

CHAPTER 22

INTER-GENERATIONAL MAGIC

FAMILIES ARE UNIQUELY positioned to not only help and support each other, but also to learn from each other. Certainly, there's the benefit you would expect of older generations setting a good example for younger generations, but the opposite can be just as true. You've probably seen examples where older adults feel younger by spending time around and learning from a younger generation. Technology is one area about which many younger family members can teach older relatives and that can be rewarding for both. Witnessing an older adult learn how to "facetime" a grandchild or great-grandchild across the country is magical.

Because genetics do play a role in our health, it's important to pass along family health history information that younger generations can benefit and learn from. Armed with information about your family's tendencies toward high blood pressure, diabetes, depression, or any health condition can give you a chance to address something early before it becomes a problem for you. I have met many people who have shared a resolve to *not* follow in their parents', grandparents', and aunts'/uncles' footsteps around something like obesity or heart disease after watching an unfortunate pattern across generations that was preventable. Breaking the chain can be a formidable and noble goal.

The "Sandwich Generation" has interesting inter-generational dynamics about wellness. As we age, if we have both parents and children, these relationships go through many phases. One of the most difficult phases can be when your parents begin to need care and you still have children that need care as well.

This so-called "sandwich" period does not happen to all people, depending on the timing of the presence and needs of parents and the presence and age of children. If you do find yourself in a situation where you are caring for both parents and children at the same time, it makes your well-being more important than ever. Embrace the fact that modest exercise along with self-care will improve your mental and physical health for the sandwich period.

Caring for aging parents is, by itself, a great opportunity for families to synergize their health habits. The feeling that you are "in this together" can bring peace while dealing with the illness, physical and cognitive changes, and death that do befall a family. Even in the healthiest of circumstances, we will all be dealing with aging and death, and it helps when our philosophies are consistent within a family. Specifically, there may come a time in every family, when we are forced to deal with difficult decisions regarding aging, whether living alone is still safe, and what kind of medical intervention we want or need. I highly recommend the book *Being Mortal* by Atul Gawande for a thought-provoking and conversation-starting look at illness, aging, and death. We would all benefit from learning how to have difficult conversations now about a loved ones' wishes, should they be unable to make medical decisions for themselves in the future.

Communication around sensitive and important issues is best when it's discussed early and often. When we wait until after a crisis happens to discuss our wishes, needs, and desired scenarios, we put ourselves at a disadvantage.

Whoever defines family for you, share with each other, laugh with each other, and support each other. Remember that two of the common characteristics of centenarians are social connectedness and putting family first. Longevity and quality relationships go hand in hand. Use this book with the people you love!

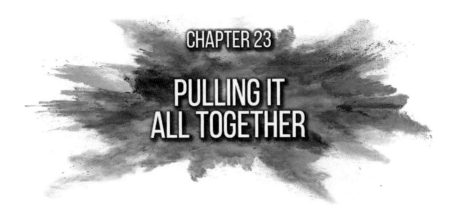

CHAPTER 23

PULLING IT ALL TOGETHER

STRONG BODY. SHARP brain. Endless energy. How far have we come in pulling together the overlapping factors and habits that help us build all three?

The concepts presented in this book were not meant to be surprising and we didn't rely on the latest research because the core recommendations don't change much from one research study to the next. As I mentioned earlier about energy specifically, good wellness habits truly resemble the philosophy of "everything I ever needed to know, I learned in kindergarten". The information makes sense. That's not the hard part. What matters is how we can ingest and successfully apply the principles in our lives for the long term.

THE KEY CONCEPTS

What are some of the important factors that impact more than one of our goals of a strong body, sharp brain, and endless energy?

- Master our mindset
- Cardiovascular exercise
- Strength training exercise

- Stretching exercise
- Move more during the day
- Don't smoke
- Eat more of the superfoods and less processed foods
- Maintain a healthy weight
- Resist fad diet
- Drink lots of water
- Get enough sleep
- Manage stress
- Maintain an active social and/or family life with meaningful relationships
- Have purposeful pursuits
- Always keep learning
- Protect your healthy hearing
- Include change, surprise, and zest in daily life

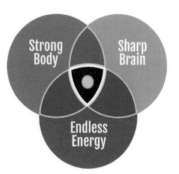

Remember, the one item that has the biggest impact on all three areas is: EXERCISE!

A LAST WORD ON MOTIVATION

As we start tying all the loose ends together, there is still the nagging awareness that many home treadmills serve as glorified clothing racks, gym memberships go unused, and healthy foods remain an afterthought. The challenge, as we have learned, is accountability. It will always be up to you. Nobody can do it for you, and nobody can take it from you. Let's recap some of the more important thoughts on this elusive thing called "motivation".

Exercise is important, but each individual exercise session will never be urgent. For it to work, it must become a priority that you schedule, protect, and treat as part of your day. Put it on your calendar like any other appointment and don't be too quick to give it up when something else comes up or someone else demands that their agenda take top priority.

Our fast-paced world is not going to cooperate in helping us find time to be more active. If it's going to happen, it's something you have to take ownership of and work at. The rest of the world is more than happy to keep heaping on the responsibilities until you say "enough".

Avoid "all or none" thinking; this includes categorizing yourself as an "exerciser" or "non-exerciser". More is better than less, but some is better than none. And some will keep the habit in place.

Habit is gold. Treat it as such.

Feel good that you are doing something for yourself and making an investment in your health.

Exercise is one thing we cannot delegate. No matter who you are or what else is on your plate, nobody can exercise for you.

When we are really honest with ourselves, we make time for the things we want to do. Period.

Free yourself from counter-productive thinking, such as comparing yourself to others.

The next year is going to come faster than you think. Do you really want to start and stop an overly stringent program a dozen times or gradually add some realistic changes to your life that you can maintain for the long haul?

WHAT ALL SUCCESSFUL LONG-TERM EXERCISERS HAVE IN COMMON

"What do they have that I don't have?" You may still be struggling to find a fitness routine that will stick. You may still be waiting for the click that turns on your internal motivation to change your habits. If you want to be successful, model your efforts after those who are being successful, right? What do they have in common?

- **SOMETHING** that acts as a common thread to string the weeks and months together.
  When a new routine is young and fragile, you'll need to find some "thing" to serve as a common thread through the weeks and months. It could be a class, an exercise buddy, a personal trainer, or a coach, for example. It doesn't matter what it is that ties the weeks together, but going it alone usually doesn't cut it.

- An activity they enjoy.
  Taking a walk can be blissful alone time. Taking an exercise class can be great social time. Bike riding with the kids can be great family time. What's going to be fun for you? Whatever it is...if it's not fun, it's no wonder you're not sticking to it.

- Flexibility. A back-up plan.
  Travel, a sick family member, and deadlines at work can all spell trouble for your exercise consistency unless you've already figured out what you'll do when obstacles arise.

- Priority. It's just what they do.
  They have the desire to "get a workout in no matter what" on a regular basis. It's not that they never skip a workout, but they feel like something is missing when they do. They get right back on it as soon as they can.

Never fear. If you don't yet have the motivational click, you can get it, all in due time. Surround yourself with the right messages and continue to do your best. Congratulations on what you are doing so far. For more tips and reflections from people like you who are making it work, check out Appendix 4. You may want to refer to it whenever you need some inspiration.

GET STARTED!

Today is a Meaningful Part of Your Life.

Someday is a dangerous word. Today is a powerful word.

It is up to you to decide how to spend the minutes that make up each day that make up your life.

It is up to you to decide what kind of attitude, attention, and priority to give to all the pieces of your life.

It is up to you to decide how you will live every today that makes up your life.

Can you feel a shift in your attitude and your confidence since Chapter 1? You know now that you can and will do something to improve your health and fitness. And you will start today! What's the next step? What have you learned through the pages of this book?

It all begins with you. Nobody can do this for you.

There is no magic wand.

Make a commitment to yourself.

Keep your focus on all the benefits you have to gain, especially the ones closest to your heart.

Anticipate the roadblocks and strategize around them.

Get a positive mindset and envision success. Picture yourself doing it!

Start slow; just getting there is the goal. The content is less important. Be happy with small steps, heading in the right direction.

Plan it into your day. Wake up thinking about when you're going to be active.

Seek support. Recruit friends and family members to join you on this journey.

Find ways to simplify your life and clear out the mental and physical clutter that bogs you down.

Strive for long-term consistency, not perfection or overnight results.

A healthy lifestyle is a work in progress.

It is a journey. There is no finish line.

Establishing the habit is more important than the content.

Once the habit is established, the content will probably grow and evolve. See what happens!

Please let me know how you are doing with gaining your stronger body, sharper brain, and endless energy. I care! Visit me at www.CathyRichards.net/BoomExtras. I'll be waiting. When you visit, you will find help, support, and accountability at your fingertips.

I wish you success, peace of mind, and happiness. I wish good health for you and your families.

My own parents, my husband, and my children have taught me many lessons along the way and none more important than valuing relationships and having the strength of body and mind to put into those relationships.

Close your eyes and picture yourself and your family members ten years from now, healthy and happy. Bring that vision to life! It's never too early and it's never too late. You can do it! What are you waiting for? It's worth it and you are worth it!

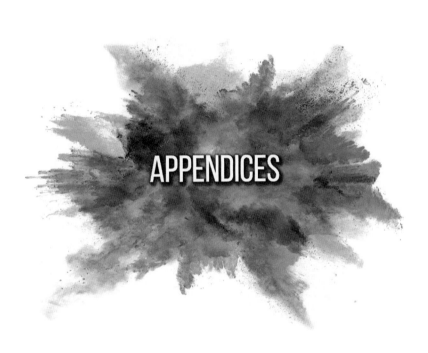

APPENDICES

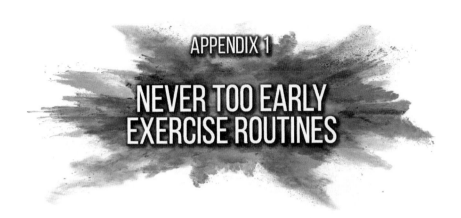

APPENDIX 1

NEVER TOO EARLY EXERCISE ROUTINES

For video clips of all of these exercises, visit www.CathyRichards.net/BoomExtras.

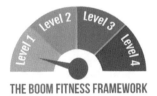

THE BOOM FITNESS FRAMEWORK

LEVEL 1: JUST MOVE

Accumulate 30 minutes of intentional movement on most days. It does not need to be all at once. It can be broken up throughout the day.

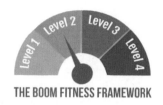

THE BOOM FITNESS FRAMEWORK

LEVEL 2: THE 20-MINUTE NO EQUIPMENT HOME EXERCISE PLAN

Frequency: 3 times per week

Your 20-minute workout will include:

- 15 minutes of cardiovascular exercise (walking or using a cardiovascular machine) followed by the standing calf stretch
- One abdominal strengthening exercise
- One upper body strengthening exercise
- One lower body strengthening exercise
- One stretching exercise—lower back stretch

CARDIOVASCULAR EXERCISE

15 minutes of walking (you can start and end right at your own front door) or another cardiovascular exercise at a moderate intensity, followed by a quick Standing Calf Stretch at the end.

Standing Calf Stretch
Stand with your feet together and take a big step backward with one foot. Next, shift your weight forward so that your front knee is bent, but the knee is not jutting out past your toes. Be sure to keep the heel of your back foot on the floor. If you don't feel a stretch in your calf of the back leg, you'll need to take a bigger step backwards with the back leg. Hold this position for about 15 seconds and then switch.

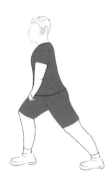

ABDOMINAL STRENGTHENING EXERCISE

Plank

Start on the floor lying on your stomach. Come up on your toes and forearms, keeping your body completely straight (don't let your hips sag down or pike up). If you find that this position is too intense, you can do the modified version on your toes and hands. The goal is to stay in this position for as long as possible. At first, this could be just ten seconds, but you will want to build up to 60 seconds or more. Once you are able to plank for more than a minute, you may be ready for more advanced abdominal strengthening exercises.

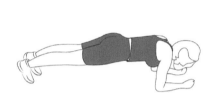
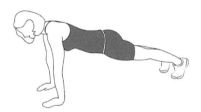

UPPER BODY STRENGTHENING EXERCISE

Push-ups

Start face down on your hands and knees or hands and feet. Be sure to keep your body rigid as you go down and up and focus on bending your elbows fully.

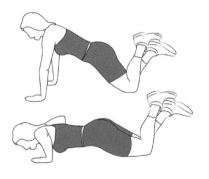

When you aren't quite strong enough to do the full range of motion correctly, your body may decide on its own to "cheat" by not letting you go down very far or not bending at the elbow. (Your body is very wise—it doesn't want you to fall on your face!). Take that as an indicator to start with a less intense version that you can perform correctly and gradually build from there. The illustration shows "modified push-ups" on your knees. If the "modified" push up is too difficult, try "wall push-ups" by standing a few feet from a wall. Place your hands on the wall at shoulder height, bend your elbows, and move your body towards and then away from the wall. If the modified version is too easy, you can do full body pushups on your toes with a straight body, but only if you can bend your elbows fully and keep your body straight while you lower completely to the floor and push back up. If an honest assessment shows that your rear end stays up while your head goes down, or you are sagging through the hips while trying to do a full body push-up, you're better off doing the modified push-up until you become stronger.

LOWER BODY STRENGTHENING EXERCISE

Stationary Lunges

Stand in a wide lunge position with your feet parallel. The front foot is planted, and the back heel is raised up so your weight is on the ball of the foot only. Slowly lower your body down until your back knee almost touches the floor while letting your front knee bend to 90 degrees. Notice how your front knee stays straight above your front foot and does not push forward. Also notice how your body from your head to your back knee stays vertical. Push straight up through the heel of your front foot and the ball of your back foot until you are up again. Do not push forward, only push up. Repeat the movement up to 10 or 20 times on one side before switching to the opposite foot in front.

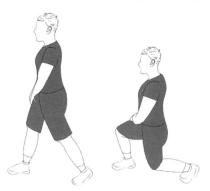

LOWER BACK STRETCH

Lying, Knees to Chest

Lie on your back and pull both knees to your chest, clasping your hands under your knees if possible. Hold this position for at least 30 seconds, or as long as several min- 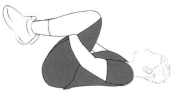 utes if you have chronic lower back pain. If you can only hold it for 30 seconds, repeat it several times.

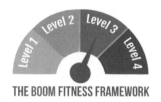

THE BOOM FITNESS FRAMEWORK

LEVEL 3: THE 40-MINUTE MINIMAL EQUIPMENT HOME EXERCISE PLAN

Frequency: 3–4 times per week

Content:

- 20 minutes of any cardiovascular exercise, 3–4 times per week (walking, jogging, elliptical machine, or stationary bicycle)
- A short (<20-minute) strength training routine, 3 times per week (one set of one exercise per muscle group using a resistance that causes fatigue between 8-15 repetitions)
- Several stretching exercises for key muscle groups

CARDIOVASCULAR EXERCISE

Upgrade your 15-minute Level 2 aerobic workout to 20 minutes at a moderate intensity.

STRENGTH TRAINING ROUTINE

1. Dumbbell Chest Press (chest)

If you are using a bench, lie on your back. If you are using an exercise ball, sit on it and then walk your feet out until you are lying on the ball as pictured. Extend your arms up directly over your chest, with your elbows straight. Slowly bring your elbows down until the inside end of each dumbbell is touching the outside of your chest/armpit area. Bring the dumbbells back up to the starting position, keeping the dumbbells straight up over your chest (don't let them drift over your face or stomach).

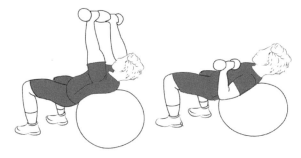

2. Seated Tubing Row (back)

Sit on the floor with your feet wider than shoulder width apart, and your knees slightly bent. Wrap the tubing around the instep portion of both shoes. (Don't try this barefoot—ouch!) Criss-cross the tubing, forming an "X", and then hold the tubing itself, as opposed to the handles. (When you hold the handles, unless you have very long arms, you'll likely find there is too much slack in the tubing, making the exercise too easy.) Pull your elbows back, being conscious to squeeze your shoulder blades together. Slowly return to the starting position.

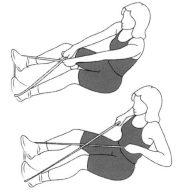

3. Dumbbell Side Raise (shoulders)

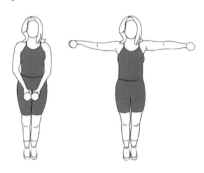

Stand, holding dumbbells in front of your body, palms facing each other. Slowly lift your arms up to the side until they are horizontal, keeping your elbows slightly bent. Your wrists should remain straight. When you reach the top, your wrists and elbows should be the same height, with your palms facing the floor. Slowly lower down to the starting position. If the dumbbells are too heavy, you won't be able to keep your elbows and wrists level, nor your palms facing down. You also want to avoid arching your back, which can happen if the dumbbells are too heavy. Think of the ending position as that of a male gymnast in the rings or imagine yourself holding a bucket in each hand. If your arms twist so that your palms no longer face the floor, you will spill your buckets of water.

4. Dumbbell Bicep Curl (biceps)

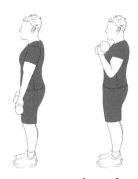

Begin with your arms at your sides with your palms facing front. Begin bending one elbow, so that when you end your palm is facing your chest in front. Return to start-ing position and then begin the other arm. To make it more challenging (and finish more quickly), you can do both arms at the same time. Regardless, be sure that your elbows always go from completely straight to completely bent and don't use momentum to swing the dumbbell up. When you lower your arm down, the temptation is to stop and start coming back up before your elbow is completely straight. That's the easy way out! Keep yourself honest by going all the way down and all the way up. If you can't go all the way down before coming back up or you start arching your back, the weight is probably too heavy.

5. Dumbbell Overhead Triceps Extension (triceps)

Hold one dumbbell overhead, as pictured. Notice that you are not holding the middle of the dumbbell, but rather, you slip the middle part between your thumb and index finger of both hands, and then grip the end of the dumbbell. Keep your elbows close to your head. Slowly bend your elbows so that the dumbbell drops low behind your head. Then, straighten your elbows again to return the dumbbell 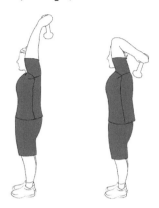 to the starting position. (When returning to the starting position, be sure that you are not moving your shoulder joints, which would throw the entire movement forward. Only move your elbow joints.)

6. Squats: Ball Squat or Dumbbell Squat (quadriceps and gluteus maximus)

The Ball Squat

Find a wall surface that is flat and bare (no door-knobs, light switches, or picture frames). Place the ball between you and the wall, about waist height, and then put your back to the ball. Press the small of your back firmly against the ball. 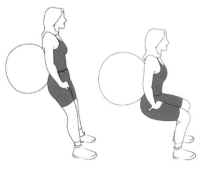 It should feel like the ball "fits" comfortably in the arch of your back. Adjust your feet so that they are about shoulder-width apart and parallel to each other. Make sure your feet are also several feet away from the wall. If your feet are too close to the wall, your knees will jut out uncomfortably once you begin the motion. If this happens to you, move your feet a few more inches away from the wall and try again. It may take a few tries to find the right foot placement for you based on your height.

The Motion
Slowly begin squatting down by bending your knees and "curling your tailbone under the ball" until your thighs are almost parallel to the floor (approaching a 90-degree bend at the knee joint). Your lower leg should remain fairly vertical, which keeps your knees over your ankles, not jutting out past your toes. Focus on keeping contact with the ball and avoid leaning forward. Once you get to the "bottom" of the range of motion, push straight up to your starting position. The ball should roll with you right back to its starting position at the small of your back.

How Far Down?
Knowing how far down to go is important and may take some practice. For some people, going all the way down to the point that their thighs are parallel to the floor is uncomfortable. You may only go half that distance and that's okay. You may find that as you build strength, you can gradually go further down. Pay attention to what your knees are telling you and only perform the exercise through the range of motion that is comfortable for you. (Note to overachievers: "Parallel" is the most advanced stopping point. It is never advisable to go past the parallel point, as that is stressful for your knee joints.)

Note: If the ball slips and starts to fall to the ground, you are performing the exercise incorrectly. Check to see if you are either leaning forward, not pressing the small of your back into the ball, and/or not curling your tailbone under the ball as you go down.

Dumbbell Squats

Stand with your feet slightly wider than shoulder-width apart. Brace the dumbbells on your shoulders as pictured. (Once you are experienced, you will probably use your heaviest dumbbells for this exercise. When you're just starting out, begin with light dumbbells or no weights at all 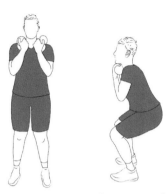 until you get the hang of it.) Slowly bend your knees and arch your back as you press your hips and butt out behind you. Try to keep your chest up. The goal is to lower down until your thighs are almost parallel to the floor without letting your knees jut out past your toes. This means that your ankle joints aren't bending at all. Once again, don't go past the parallel point. When you start coming back up, thrust your hips forward in a subtle way so that your body is straight once again.

> *A Few Words of Caution about Squats*
> Stop if you feel pain, especially in your knees. You may want to double check to make sure you are using the correct form. But even performed correctly, squats may not be for you. Listen to your body and if it hurts, don't do it.

7. Ball Hamstring Curl (hamstrings)

This is a fun exercise that may take a little practice at first in order to keep your balance! Lie on the floor on your back with your calves and ankles propped up on the ball. If the ball is too close to you (under your knees), you won't have enough room to let the ball roll. If the ball is too far away from you (under your ankles and feet only), it will probably slip

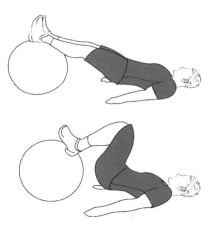

away. Brace yourself with your arms pressing down on the floor and lift up your hips. (This is where you may need to practice your balance!) Keeping your hips elevated, dig your heels into the ball, and roll the ball toward your rear end, then roll back out. You may need to occasionally reposition your feet if the ball starts slipping away from you.

8. Inner Thigh Ball Squeeze (adductors/inner thigh)

Approach the ball from behind and carefully sit on it. Roll forward slightly until your hip joint is completely straight. (Your knees are pointing down, not forward, and your feet are behind you.) If you fall off the front of the ball, try again but this time, start farther back. Once

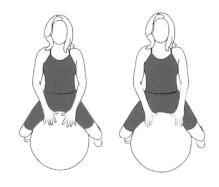

you're in a comfortable position, simply squeeze the ball with your thighs and release. I like to finish with an extended squeeze of 10 or more seconds.

9. Lying Hip Abduction with Tubing (abductors/hips)

Lie on your back on the floor, with the tubing around your feet. Be sure that the tubing is securely caught in the notch of your shoe at the instep. Your legs are overhead, but angled down a bit (not straight up), and your knees are slightly bent. You'll want about 6-10 inches of tubing between your feet. If you 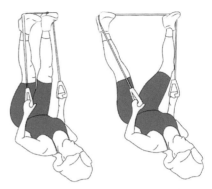 feel any cramping in your hip muscles, try angling your legs down even farther. Open and close your legs from the hip joint. Each time you press out, the tubing will stretch and apply a resistance to your hip muscles doing the work. Press out and release back in as many times as you can.

10. Plank (abdominals)

Start on the floor lying on your stomach. Come up on your toes and forearms, keeping your body completely straight (don't let your hips sag down or pike up). If you find that this position is too intense, you can do the modified version on your toes and hands. The goal is to stay in this position for as long as possible. At first, this could be just ten seconds, but you will want to build up to 60 seconds or more. Once you are able to plank for more than a minute, you may be ready for more advanced abdominal strengthening exercises.

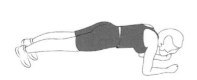
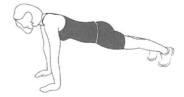

Four Key Stretches

A great way to finish off your Level 3 exercise routine is with a few stretches for those major muscle groups most in need of some TLC after a workout. There are four stretches in this level. You can hold each stretch for as little as 10–15 seconds for a quick stretch, up to 30 seconds when you're relaxing a little more into the stretch, or as long as a minute or two when you are nursing a problem in that area. Remember not to bounce.

1. Quadriceps Stretch

Stand on one foot and hold the other foot up behind you as pictured. Be sure to keep your knees close together.

2. Chest Stretch

Let your arms fall open wide. Pull your arms back, squeezing shoulder blades together.

3. Lower Back Stretch

Lie on your back and hold both knees to your chest, clasping your hands under your knees if possible. Hold this position for at least 30 seconds, or as long as several minutes if you have chronic lower back pain. If you can only hold it for 30 seconds, repeat it several times.

4. Hamstring Stretch

While lying on the floor on your back, keep one leg bent with your foot flat on the floor. Extend the other leg up and pull towards your body with your hands, keeping your knee slightly bent and your lower back pressed to the floor. Switch.

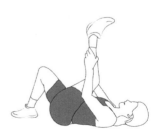

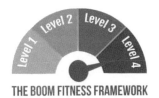

THE BOOM FITNESS FRAMEWORK

LEVEL 4: THE 60-MINUTE+ FULL-FLEDGED EXERCISE PLAN

Frequency: 3–6 times per week

Content:
- 20–60 minutes of varied aerobic exercise at a moderate intensity, 3–5 times per week (walking, jogging, step aerobics, elliptical machine, or stationary bicycle).
- A 20–40-minute weight-training routine, 3 times per week (2–3 sets per muscle group using a resistance that causes fatigue between 8-15 repetitions).
- Stretching exercises for each major muscle group.

Get professional guidance!

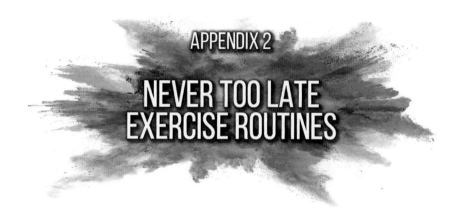

APPENDIX 2

NEVER TOO LATE EXERCISE ROUTINES

For video clips of all of these exercises, visit
www.CathyRichards.net/BoomExtras.

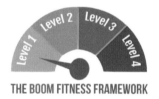

THE BOOM FITNESS FRAMEWORK

LEVEL 1: JUST MOVE

Accumulate 30 minutes of intentional movement on most days. It does not need to be all at once. It can be broken up throughout the day.

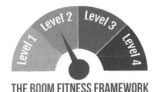

THE BOOM FITNESS FRAMEWORK

LEVEL 2: THE 20-MINUTE NO EQUIPMENT HOME EXERCISE PLAN

Frequency: 3 times per week

Your 20-minute workout will include:

- 15 minutes of cardiovascular exercise (walking or using a cardiovascular machine) followed by the standing calf stretch
- One abdominal strengthening exercise
- One upper body strengthening exercise
- One lower body strengthening exercise
- One stretching exercise

CARDIOVASCULAR EXERCISE

15 minutes of walking (you can start and end right at your own front door) or another cardiovascular exercise at a moderate intensity, followed by a quick Standing Calf Stretch at the end.

Standing Calf Stretch
Stand with your feet together and take a big step backward with one foot. Next, shift your weight forward so that your front knee is bent, but the knee is not jutting out past your toes. Be sure to keep the heel of your back foot on the floor. If you don't feel a stretch in your calf of the back leg, you'll need to take a bigger step backwards with the back leg. Hold this position for about 15 seconds and then switch.

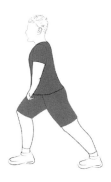

ABDOMINAL STRENGTHENING EXERCISE

Seated Abdominal Crunch

This abdominal exercise is ideal if you are not comfortable getting on the floor. In the starting position, you are sitting at the edge of the chair. Slowly lean back until you almost touch your shoulder blades to the back of the chair. You should feel your abdominal muscles tighten. Then slowly come back up to the starting position. Perform 5-20 repetitions as comfortable.

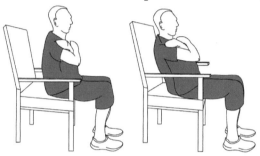

UPPER BODY STRENGTHENING EXERCISE

Seated Press Ups

Start off seated with your hands on the arms of the chair and your feet flat on the floor. Press up on your hands until your elbows are straight. Do not use your legs to help. You will not end up standing up fully. Bend your elbows to lower your body back to the chair. Perform 5-20 repetitions as comfortable.

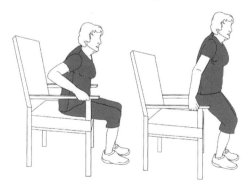

LOWER BODY STRENGTHENING EXERCISE

The Sit-to-Stand or Leg Extension

The Sit-to-Stand

Begin by sitting close to the end of a sturdy chair. Lean forward and stand up and sit back down without using your arms to assist. Perform 2-20 repetitions as you are able.

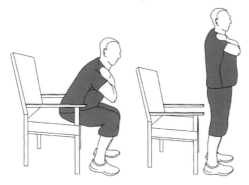

The Leg Extension

The Leg Extension is for you if you are unable to perform the sit-to-stand for even one repetition. Sit upright in a chair and lift one leg so that the knee is a bit higher than the other leg. Kick out your foot until your knee is straight and then bend it to return to the starting position. If you don't keep your moving knee a bit higher than the stationary knee, your foot will bump into the floor and stop your range of motion before you fully return to the starting position. Perform 8-12 repetitions for each leg.

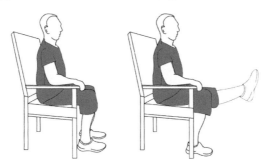

STRETCHING EXERCISE

Lower Back Stretch

While seated, place your feet shoulder-width apart, round your back over, and let your head and hands lower down. Stay in this position for 15-30 seconds. Your lower back muscles will relax and lengthen. If you have osteoporosis, lean forward with a straight spine while keeping your hands on your thighs and do not lower your head below your knees.

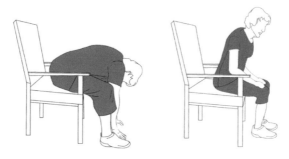

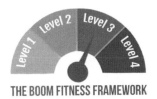

THE BOOM FITNESS FRAMEWORK

LEVEL 3: THE 40-MINUTE MINIMAL EQUIPMENT HOME EXERCISE PLAN

Frequency: 3–4 times per week

Content:

- 20 minutes of any cardiovascular exercise, 3–4 times per week (walking, jogging, elliptical machine, or stationary bicycle) followed by the standing calf stretch.

- A short (<20-minute) strength training routine, 3 times per week (one set of one exercise per muscle group using a resistance that causes fatigue between 8-15 repetitions)

- Several stretching exercises for key muscle groups

CARDIOVASCULAR EXERCISE

Upgrade your 15-minute Level 2 aerobic workout to 20 minutes at a moderate intensity. The same cautions exist for cardiovascular exercise as with the Level 2. Walking is still a great choice, as are non-impact options such as aquatic exercise, a seated elliptical machine, recumbent stationary bicycle, or a NuStep® machine.

STRENGTH TRAINING ROUTINE

1. Seated Chest Press

Wrap the exercise band behind your back and grip it on each side under your armpits. Press out in front of you until your elbows are almost straight. Slowly return to starting position and repeat.

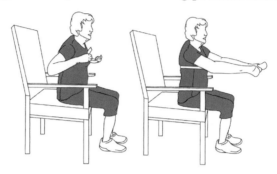

2. Seated Row

Sit upright close to the edge of the chair with your legs extended a bit, heels anchored to the floor and knees slightly bent. Wrap the exercise band around your feet, crisscross the band, and then hold one end in each hand. (Be sure that the band is anchored securely around the instep of your shoe. Do not let the band slide up towards your toes as it could slip off and ricochet towards your face!) Pull on the band, squeezing your shoulder blades together. Slowly return to starting position and repeat.

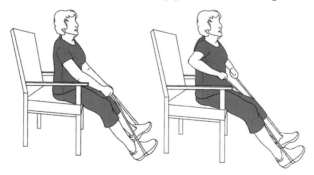

3. Biceps Curl

Sit with feet firmly planted on the floor in front of you. Anchor the band securely under your feet and grip firmly with each hand. Keeping your elbows by your side, bend your elbows ending with your palms near your shoulders. Slowly return to starting position and repeat.

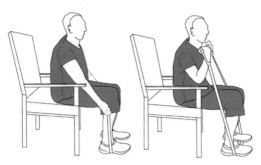

4. Triceps Extension

Grip the band with both hands in front of you, leaving 8-12 inches of band between your hands. Anchor one hand right above the chest. With the other arm, extend the elbow until your arm is straight out to the side. Slowly return to starting position and repeat.

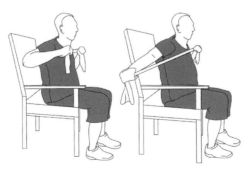

5. Seated Abdominal Crunch

Sit upright close to the edge of the chair and cross your arms over your chest. Slowly lean back until your shoulder blades barely touch the back of the chair. Hold for just a small moment, then slowly return to the starting position and repeat.

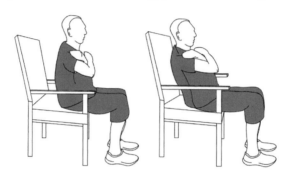

6. Leg Press

Sitting upright, lift one leg, wrap the band around the bottom of your shoe, and grip firmly in each hand. Press your foot out until the knee is almost straight. Slowly return to starting position and repeat. Switch to the other leg when finished.

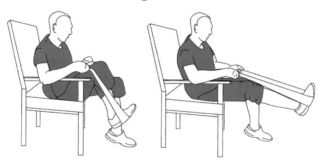

7. Ankle Circles and Point/Flex

While seated, extend one leg out and slowly circle your ankle joint, creating as big of a range of motion as possible with your toes. Do several revolutions in each direction. Then point and flex your ankle by pulling your toes firmly toward your shin and then pointing your toes away from you as firmly as possible. Repeat several times.

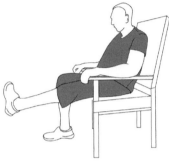

8. Side Leg Lift

Standing at a wall or holding on to a chair, lift your leg out to the side. Keep your posture straight and do not lean over to the opposite side as you lift the leg. You should only be able to lift it a small amount. Lower the leg but do not let it touch the floor before lifting again (unless you really need to). Switch to the other leg.

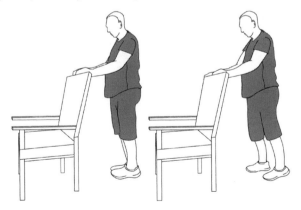

9. Standing Calf Raise

Stand on both feet at a wall or holding on to a chair. Slowly rise up on your toes and then lower back down. For a higher intensity version and if your balance is very good, stand on one foot with the non-weight bearing foot propped behind the other ankle. If performing the one-leg version, you will need to switch to the other leg when you are done.

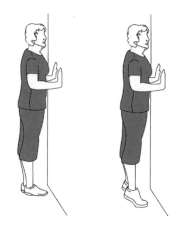

10. Chin Tuck

Seated or standing, pull your chin back towards you and hold for 5-10 seconds. Repeat. When you release, try not to release fully to the point that your head started at, as we all tend to carry our heads too far forward, which throws our body alignment off.

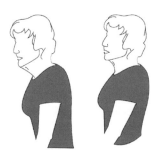

Four Key Stretches

1. Seated Chest Stretch

Let your arms fall open wide. Pull your arms back, squeezing your shoulder blades together.

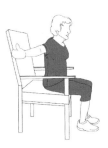

2. Seated Lower Back Stretch

While seated close to the end of the chair, place your feet shoulder-width apart, round your back over, and let your head and hands lower down. If you have osteoporosis, lean forward with a straight spine and support your weight with your hands on your thighs.

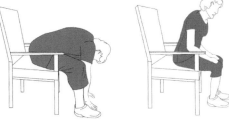

3. Seated Hamstring Stretch

Sit close to the end of the chair with one leg straight out in front of you on your heel. Gently lean forward towards the straight leg.

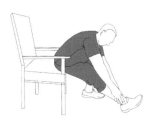

4. Neck Stretch

Seated or standing, gently tilt your ear towards your shoulder. To deepen the stretch, you can gently pull on your head and also extend the opposite arm out to the side. Switch.

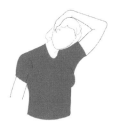

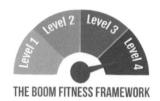

THE BOOM FITNESS FRAMEWORK

LEVEL 4: THE 60-MINUTE+ FULL-FLEDGED EXERCISE PLAN

Frequency: 3–6 times per week

Content:

- 20–60 minutes of varied aerobic exercise at a moderate intensity, 3–5 times per week (walking, aquatic exercise, seated elliptical, recumbent stationary bicycle, etc.).
- A 20–40-minute weight-training routine, 3 times per week (2–3 sets per muscle group using a resistance that causes fatigue between 8-15 repetitions).
- Stretching exercises for each major muscle group.

Get professional guidance!

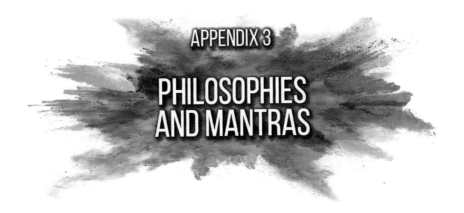

APPENDIX 3

PHILOSOPHIES AND MANTRAS

My challenge to you is attitude. This is a long-term process. It's a choice, a priority, and a lifestyle. It's about forever. There is no finish line. It's all about making small changes little by little that you have no intention of ever stopping. They will slowly add up.

Visualization is a powerful thing. You must picture success—you have to be able to SEE it, feel it, and already be there in your mind. Live as if you are already there. Think as if you are already there.

Exercise has more far-reaching benefits in more categories of your life than any other single thing you can do.

It's never too early and it's never too late.

More might be better than less, but some is better than none.

Done is better than perfect, especially when perfect prevents actions.

Habit is more important than content.

Exercise is one thing that cannot be delegated. Nobody can do this for you but you!

You can't afford not to!

Successful people do what unsuccessful people just don't like to do.

The only thing that often separates successful people from non-successful people is ACTION.

What you focus on grows. Think positive always!

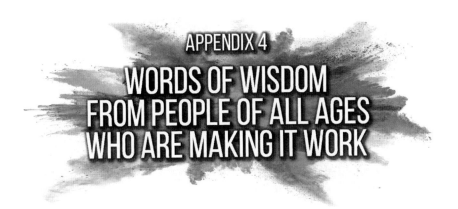

APPENDIX 4
WORDS OF WISDOM FROM PEOPLE OF ALL AGES WHO ARE MAKING IT WORK

WHAT DO THEY **have that I don't have?**

You may still be struggling to find the right mix of habits that work for you to have a strong body, sharp brain, and endless energy. Why not pick up a few pointers from those who are successful in what you are striving for? There may be something in the following collection that really speaks to you.

Over the years, I've learned that a lot of motivated, goal-oriented people are oftentimes their own worst critics, which is detrimental to their health and fitness. After realizing I was magnifying my flaws and having negative self-talk, I decided enough was enough. I shifted my goals to be focused on actions within my control (i.e. exercising three times a week, adding a green veggie to every meal) rather than giving so much power to numbers on a scale. My small accomplishments every week built momentum for more healthy habits and the framework for what is now my lifestyle.

—Maria Bross, age 29, Charleston, SC

Each day is an opportunity to develop into a better version of yourself. Focus on what's working. Upgrade the quality of your thoughts. Never give up!

—Peter Colwell, age 44, Germantown, MD

1. After dinner, make a habit to walk for 20 minutes. This transition makes you stop eating and gets you moving. It also helps stabilize blood sugar throughout the rest of the night and into the morning, so you will feel better.

2. Cook two big, healthy meals on Sunday. That way you are set up for success for the week. Not only will you be doing fewer dishes in the week, you'll have more mental energy to focus on other things besides dinner. It can be something simple that tastes better as a leftover. We just made black eyed peas with ground turkey, corn, and Swiss chard. It's delicious! The Instant pot can also save you time.

3. Pasture-raised eggs and healthy fats are your friend. Don't be afraid of either. Cook with olive oil for low heat, and avocado oil or coconut oil for high heat. Choose pasture-raised eggs because they have more omega-3. Stay away from vegetable oil—it's too high in omega-6 fatty acids and is processed poorly.

4. Limit sugar.

5. Swap out white rice for red lentils in any recipe. It's high in protein and fiber. It cooks quickly! Add them to boiling water for 10 minutes and drain them when they are ready to be added to any stir fry or bulk up any meal to make it go further. They are very cheap, too.

—Laura Cotton, age 35, Austin, TX (registered dietitian)

Be kind to yourself. Take one step out of your comfort zone each day. Be playful.

—Nicolette Stearns, midlife, Germantown, MD

Love playing tennis—great exercise, social time, and a fun way to work out!

—Ellen Robin, soon-to-be empty nester, Germantown, MD

I attribute my quick recovery from three major surgeries to being in good condition—even if it wasn't enough to prevent the most recent surgery. Many experienced hospital folks told me the recovery would be strong because of that conditioning. I quickly became determined to focus on what was possible with recovery rather than what had happened. I attribute much of that readiness to my lifetime habit of fitness and my familiarity with what is possible with exercise.

—Dan Kolar, age 63, Damascus, MD

Over the past twenty years, my Team and I at Masterpiece Living have worked with tens of thousands of older adults to help them modify their lifestyle in order to age in a better way. The most significant thing we've learned is that change should be in very small steps. This allows us to succeed and for the change to be durable.

—Roger Landry MD MPH President, Masterpiece Living

I am a health coach and geriatric occupational therapist who is all too familiar with the pitfalls of aging. Most chronic diseases are treatable and preventable. The way I stay on track is by living the way humans were designed to live: a mostly plant-based diet, daily movement, socialization, and sleep.

—Sue Paul, www.suempaul.com

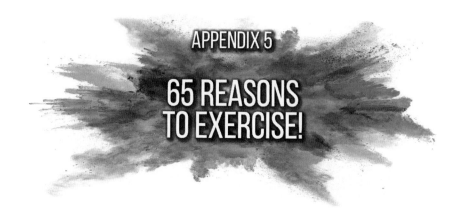

APPENDIX 5

65 REASONS TO EXERCISE!

1. Exercise burns 2–12 times as many calories per minute as sitting.

2. Exercise can help reduce the amount of fat on your body.

3. Exercise increases your muscle mass.

4. Exercise improves the strength and endurance of your existing muscle mass.

5. Exercise helps fight fatigue.

6. Exercise just makes you feel better!

7. Nobody else is going to do it for you.

8. Exercise gives you more energy.

9. Exercise gives you a more positive attitude.

10. Exercise gives you more confidence in your ability to accomplish goals.

11. Exercise success translates into mental fortitude for other challenges in life.

12. Exercise increases your body confidence.

13. Exercise improves your sex life.

14. Exercise reduces symptoms of PMS.

15. Exercise increases your bone density, decreasing your risk of osteoporosis.

16. Exercise lubricates your joints to supply more nutrients for healthier cartilage tissue.

17. Exercise can prevent constipation.

18. Exercise helps your body better regulate insulin and blood sugar levels.

19. Exercise reduces your risk of diabetes.

20. Exercise increases anti-inflammatory hormones, which may help prevent some forms of cancer.

21. Exercise reduces your risk of cardiovascular disease.

22. Exercise reduces high blood pressure.

23. Exercise can reduce total cholesterol.

24. Exercise can help increase HDL cholesterol (the good kind).

25. You've got to use it or lose it.

26. Exercise increases your resting metabolic rate.

27. Exercise increases your metabolic rate during all of your daily activities.

28. Exercise helps you perform the activities of daily life with less strain.

29. Exercise improves the flexibility of your muscles and joints.

30. Exercise helps improve your balance.

31. Exercise helps improve your posture.

32. Exercise helps reduce lower back pain.

33. Exercise improves your self-esteem.

34. Exercise reduces depression.

35. Exercise reduces anxiety.

36. Exercise reduces stress.

37. Exercise reduces absenteeism at work or school.

38. Exercise helps you spend less in health care costs.

39. Exercise helps you concentrate better.

40. Exercise helps you work more efficiently.

41. Exercise helps you sleep better.

42. Exercise makes your heart stronger.

43. Exercise makes your lungs stronger and increases your oxygen capacity.

44. Exercise increases your cardiovascular endurance.

45. Exercise helps your clothes fit better.

46. Because your doctor wants you to!

47. Exercise enhances overall function of the brain and nerves.

48. Exercise helps keep you strong as you age.

49. Exercise promotes your independence as you age.

50. You'll always be able to carry in your own groceries.

51. Exercise helps you recover from surgery faster.

52. Exercise helps symptoms of arthritis (except during an acute inflammation).

53. Exercise strengthens your immune system, helping you fight off colds and flu.

54. Exercise helps you keep up with your kids and grandkids.

55. Exercise helps relieve headaches.

56. Exercise makes it easier to go up and down the stairs without getting out of breath.

57. Exercise eases lots of miscellaneous aches and pains.

58. Exercise is something you can do to have time for yourself.

59. Exercise gives you a natural high.

60. Exercise makes you want to eat healthier.

61. Exercise helps you feel young.

62. Exercise helps you feel like exercising some more!

63. Exercise helps you clear your head.

64. Exercise reduces your risk of falling.

65. Exercise is a great way to do something for yourself that no one else can do!

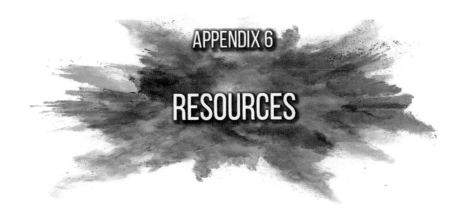

APPENDIX 6

RESOURCES

Recommended Reading

Age Wave, Ken Dychtwald

Being Mortal, Atul Gawande

The Blue Zones, Dan Buettner

The Brain that Changes Itself, Norman Doidge

Emotional Agility: Get Unstuck, Embrace Change, and Thrive in Work and Life, Susan David

Live Long, Die Short, Roger Landry

Nutrition Action Healthletter (www.nutritionaction.com)

Resilient Leadership, Bob Duggan and Jim Moyer

Spell Success in Your Life, Peter Colwell

Successful Aging, John W. Rowe and Robert L. Kahn

The Tipping Point, Malcom Gladwell

Other Recommended Resources

My Fitness Pal (www.myfitnesspal.com)

Fitbit (www.fitbit.com)

American College of Sports Medicine (www.acsm.org)

Senior Fitness Association (www.seniorfitness.net)

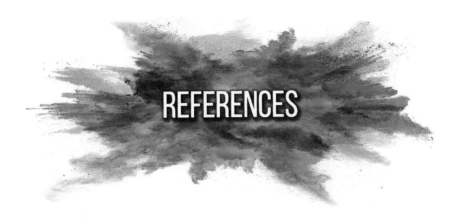

REFERENCES

1. John W. Rowe and Robert L. Kahn, *Successful Aging*, (New York: Dell, 1998)

2. Dan Buettner, *Blue Zones*, (Washington, D.C., The National Geographic Society, 2008)

3. Gries, Kevin, Raue, Ulrika, Perkins, Ryan K., Lavin, Kaleen M., Overstreet, Brittany S., et al, "Cardiovascular and skeletal muscle health with lifelong exercise", *Journal of Applied Physiology*, Nov. 26, 2018. https://doi.org/10.1152/japplphysiol.00174.2018

4. www.GrowingBolder.com

5. Center for Disease Control and Prevention, www.CDC.gov

6. Bravata, Dena, "Using Pedometers to Increase Physical Activity and Improve Health: A Systematic Review, *JAMA*, 2007:298 (19):2296-2304

7. www.hearinghealthfoundation.org

8. American College of Sports Medicine. *ACSM's Guidelines for Exercise Testing and Prescription*, Tenth Edition, 2018. Philadelphia, PA: Lippincott Williams & Wilkins.

9. www.HHS.gov – Physical Activity Guidelines for Americans, 2018

10. www.ihrsa.org

11. www.nutritionaction.com

12. National Sleep Foundation, www.sleepfoundation.org

13. Atul Gawande, *Being Mortal: Medicine and What Matters in the End*, (New York: Metropolitan Books, Henry Hold and Company, 2014)

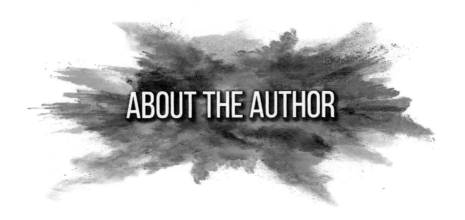

ABOUT THE AUTHOR

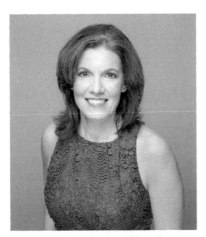

CATHY RICHARDS, M.A., owner of Inspiring Vitality, is a lifestyle and wellness strategist and speaker who helps individuals and organizations maximize physical health, brain function, and energy levels. Cathy earned the C. Everett Koop National Health Award for Worksite Health Promotion while spending the first 15 years of her career in corporate wellness for Marriott International, Inc. She then spent eight years in wellness for older adults with Asbury, the 15th largest not-for-profit continuing care retirement community in the U.S. Merging those two experiences led to Cathy's unique "never too early, never too late" approach. With a M.A. Degree in Exercise Physiology, a B.S. Degree in Kinesiological Sciences and over 20 years as a wellness coach, Cathy unlocks key mindset shifts and strategies for lasting motivation and lifestyle change at any age. Her certifications include ACSM Certified Exercise Physiologist, Wellcoaches Certified Fitness Coach, Senior Fitness Association Certified Senior Fitness Instructor, Long Term Care Instructor, and Brain Fitness Facilitator. While her children were younger, she authored *The Busy Mom's Ultimate Fitness Guide: Get Motivated and Find the Solution that Works for You!*, sharing her contagious passion for healthy living. She has been featured on numerous TV news stations and print publications including the *Washington Post*. She has presented at industry conferences and delivered motivational keynotes for business conferences, executive retreats, and senior living organizations. You can find out more about her at www.CathyRichards.net

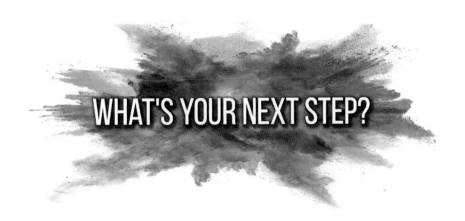

WHAT'S YOUR NEXT STEP?

YOU ARE WELL on your way to a longer, healthier life through a Strong Body, Sharp Brain, and Endless Energy! What are you going to do to incorporate this information into your daily life to make it stick? Remember one of our most important meanings of BOOM: Consider it DONE. Action and success is a foregone conclusion!

Visit Me

Visit me at www.CathyRichards.Net/BoomExtras for resources and support tailored just for those who are motivated to find and keep more vitality in their life at any age. Here are just a few of the things you'll find:

- Free downloadable extras, such as additional exercise lists, recipes, articles of interest, and much more.
- An opportunity to connect with me and with others who have similar goals. There will be group phone coaching sessions, webinars, and much more!

Submit a Review of *BOOM* on Amazon.com

Did you find value in BOOM? I hope so! If you'd like to leave an honest review on Amazon.com, I'd be very appreciative. A high volume of Amazon reviews helps an author's ranking so thank you in advance if you are so inclined. (Note that Amazon allows you to leave a review even if you did not obtain your copy of *BOOM* from Amazon.)

Keynotes and Workshops

Does your group or organization have an upcoming meeting that needs an energy boost and some great content? Contact me at www.CathyRichards.net/speaking for more information on speaking engagements. I'd love to come speak to your group!

Social Media

I would love to stay in touch via social media. You can follow me here:

YouTube: www.cathyrichards.net/YouTube

FaceBook: @InspiringVitality
(www.facebook.com/InspiringVitality)

Instagram: @InspiringVitality
(www.Instagram.com/InspiringVitality)

LinkedIn: www.linkedin.com/in/cathymrichards

Twitter: @CRichVitality

Here's wishing you a lifetime of wellness!